Prediction of Maternal and Fetal Syndrome of Preeclampsia

Edited by Nidhi Sharma

Published in London, United Kingdom

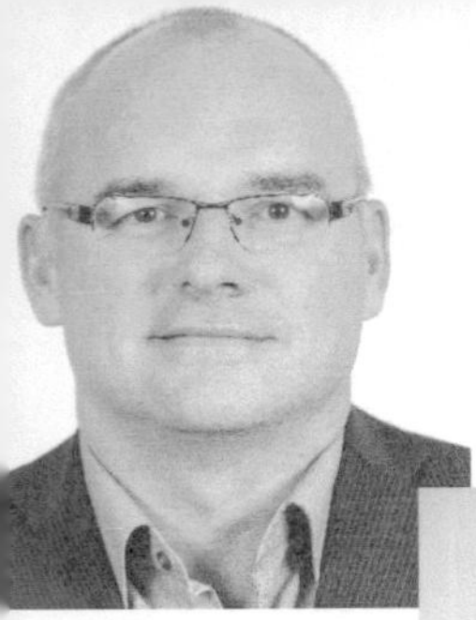
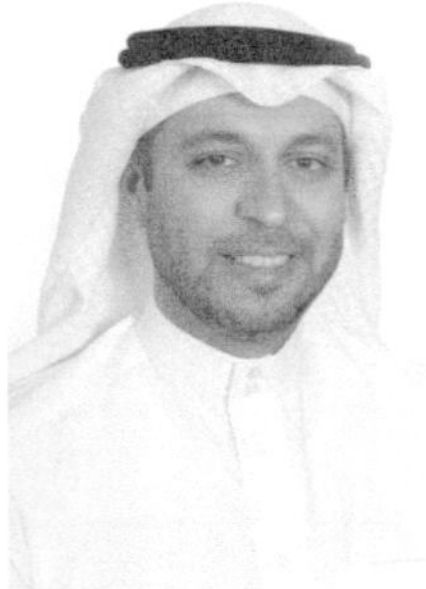
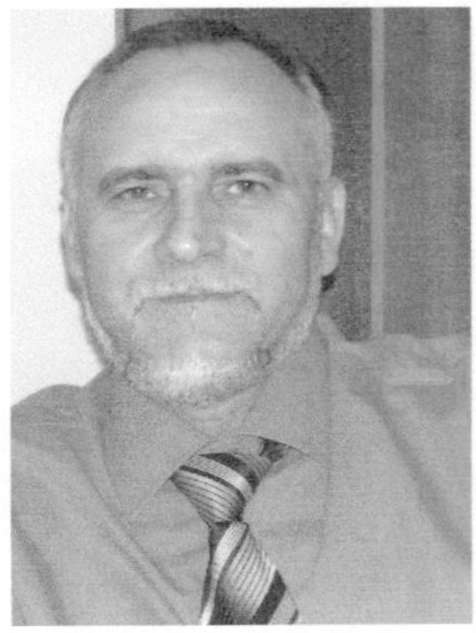
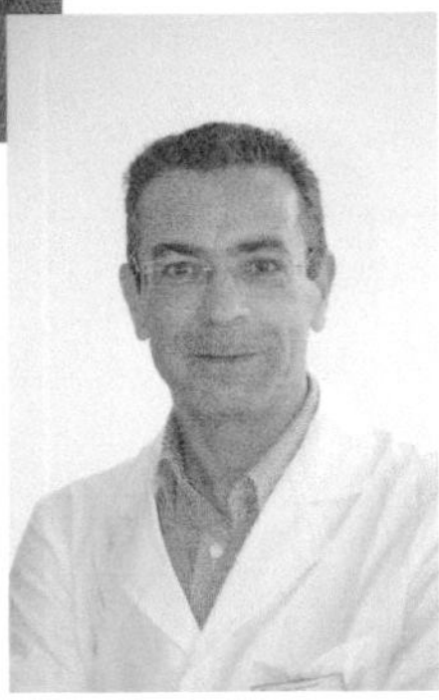
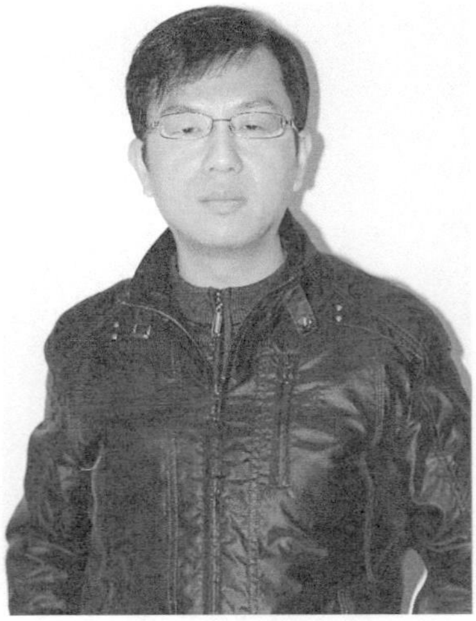
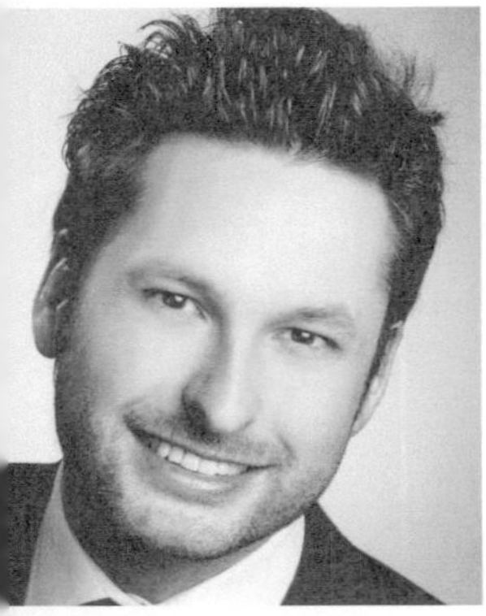
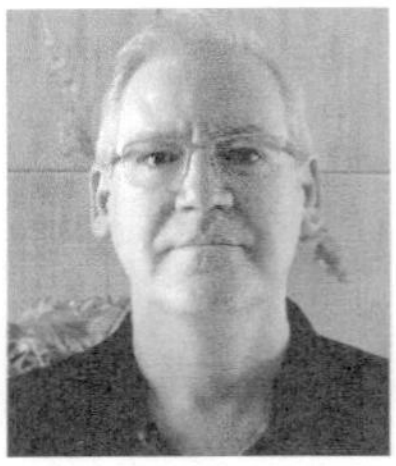

IntechOpen

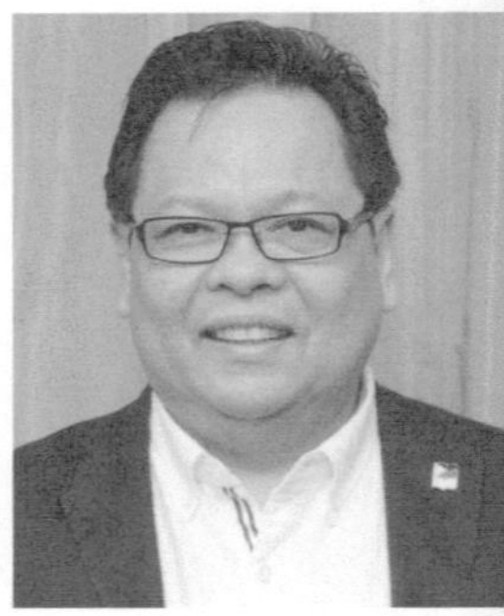
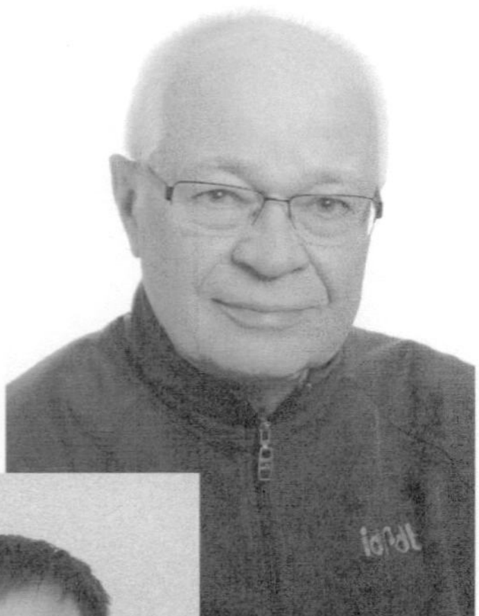
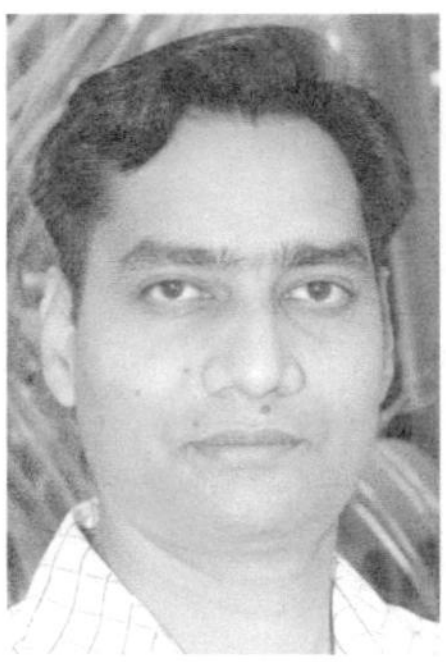
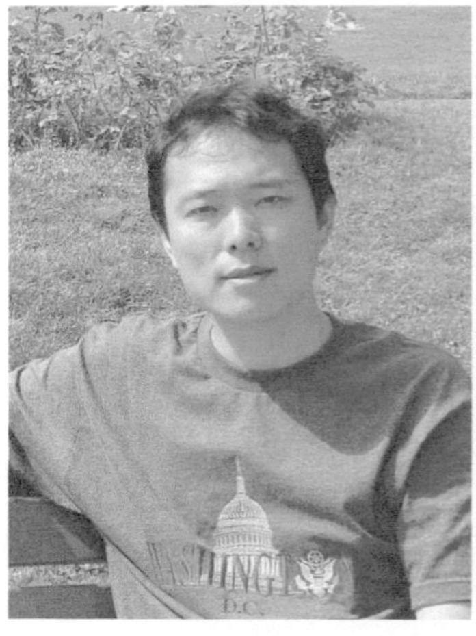
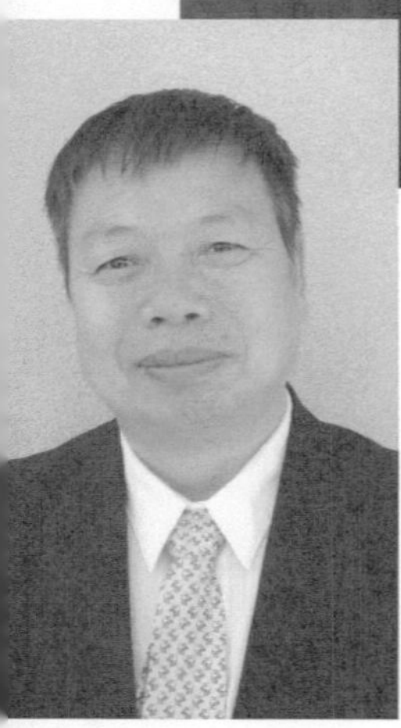
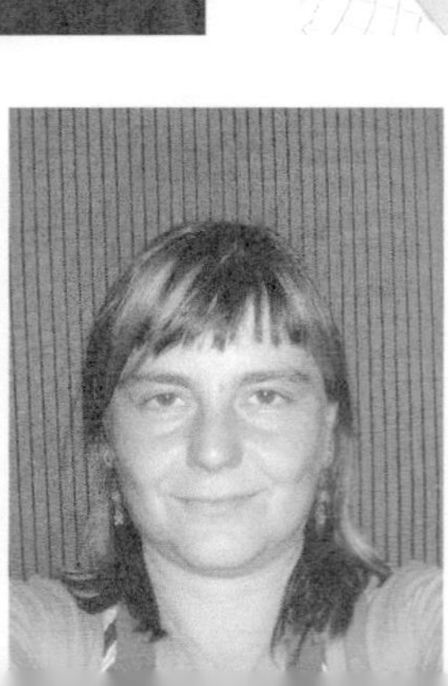

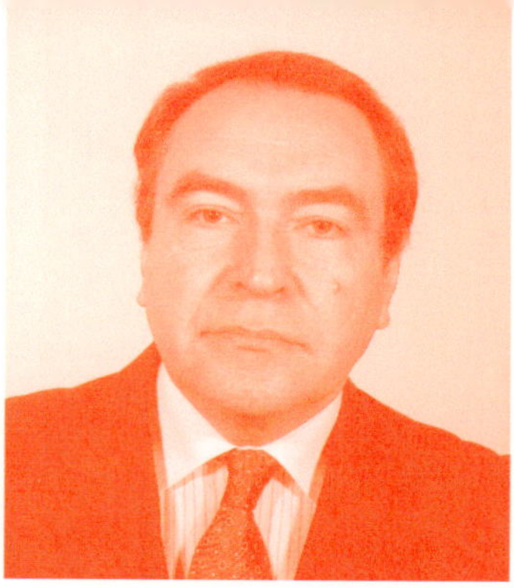

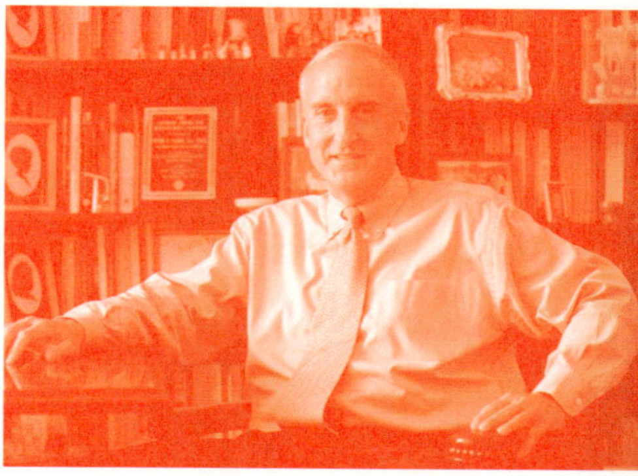

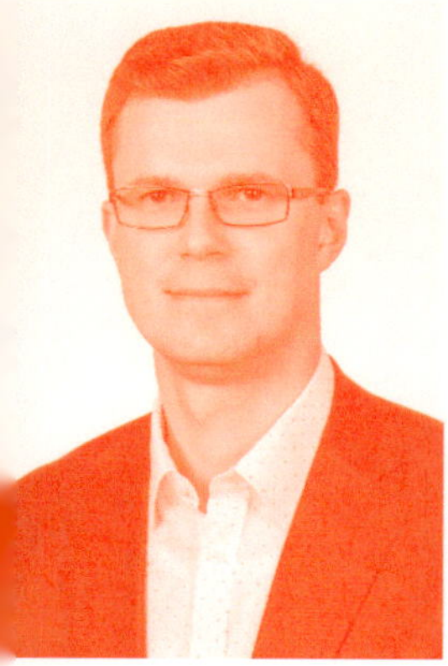

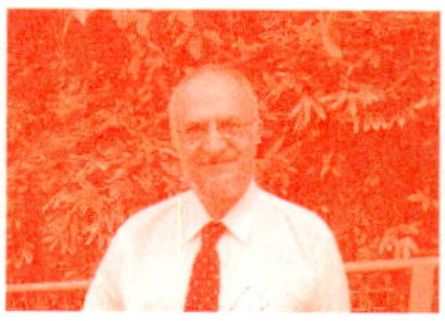

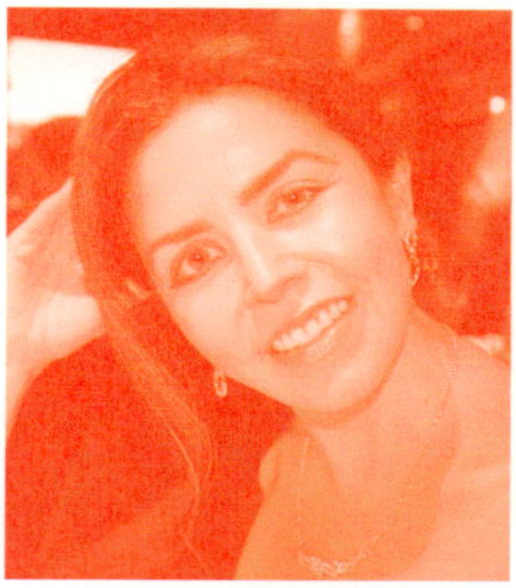

Supporting open minds since 2005

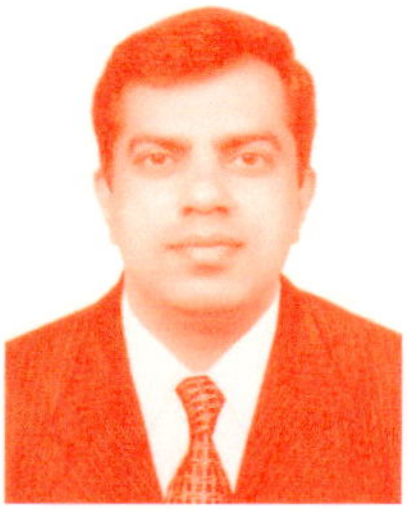

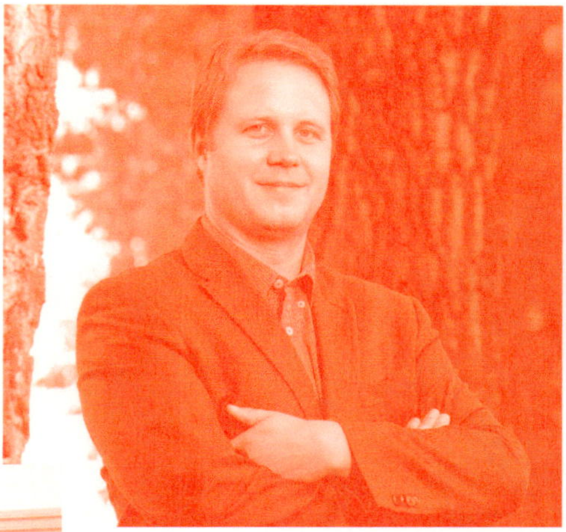

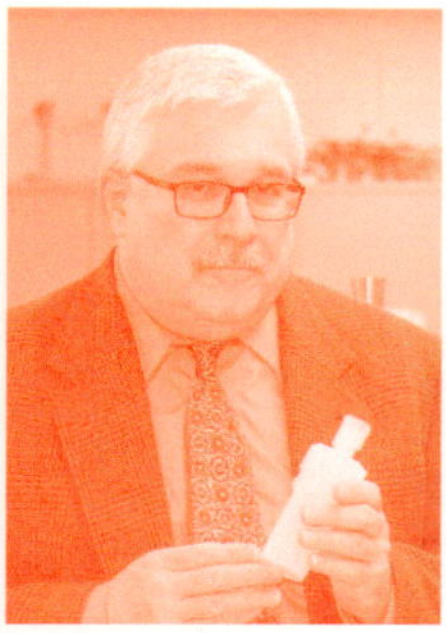

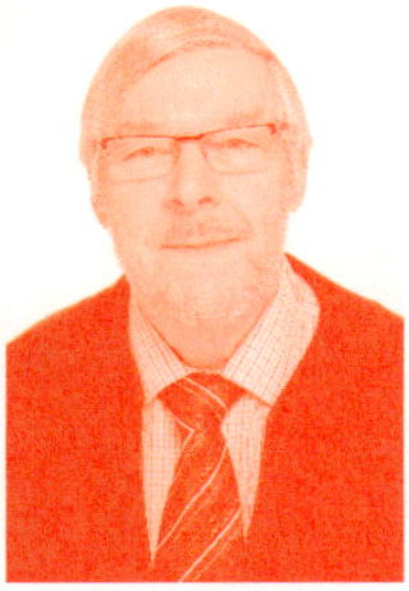

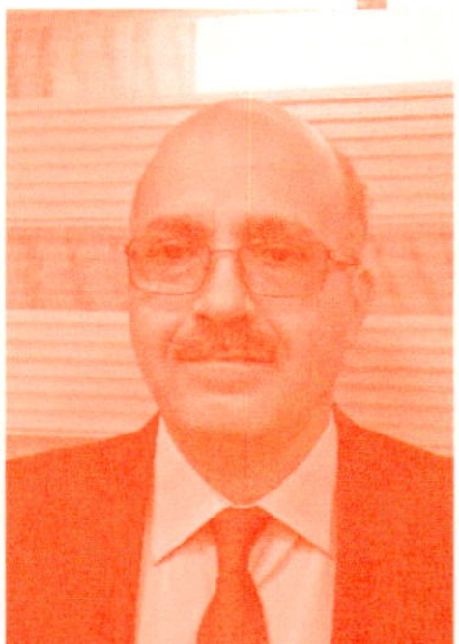

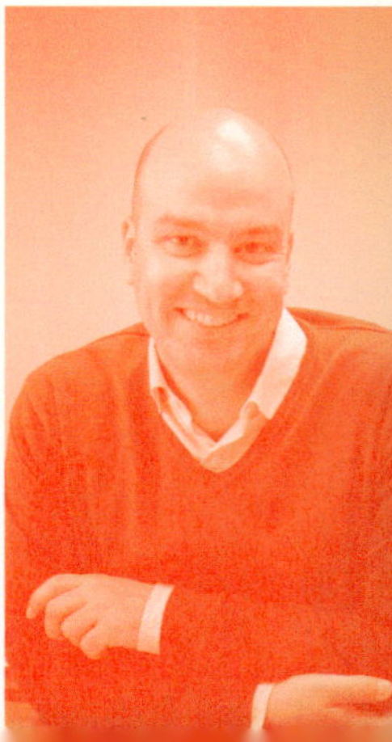

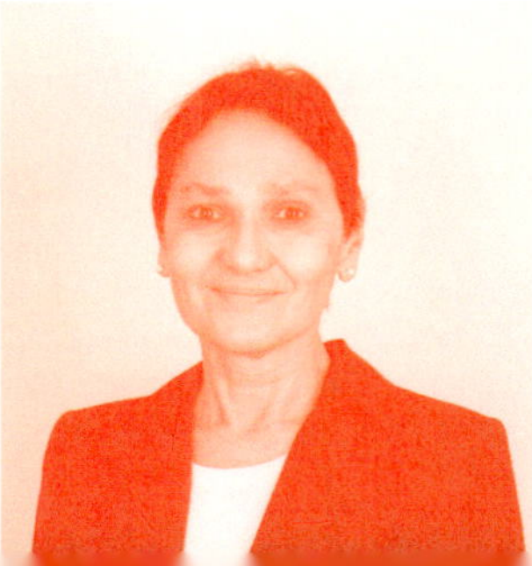

Prediction of Maternal and Fetal Syndrome of Preeclampsia
http://dx.doi.org/10.5772/intechopen.78845
Edited by Nidhi Sharma

Contributors
Joško Osredkar, Kristina Kumer, Priscila Nunes, Leandro Oliveira, Maria Terezinha Peraçoli, Mariana Romão-Veiga, Megha Karemore, Byron Baron, Maria Portelli, Sarah Ahmed, Sergio Rosales-Ortiz, Mario Borbolla-Ramos, Olivia Sanchez-Rodriguez, Karen D Garcia-Perez, Makmur Sitepu, Nidhi Sharma

First published in London, United Kingdom, 2019 by IntechOpen
IntechOpen is the global imprint of INTECHOPEN LIMITED, registered in England and Wales, registration number: 11086078, The Shard, 25th floor, 32 London Bridge Street
London, SE19SG - United Kingdom
Printed in Croatia

British Library Cataloguing-in-Publication Data
A catalogue record for this book is available from the British Library

Additional hard and PDF copies can be obtained from orders@intechopen.com

Prediction of Maternal and Fetal Syndrome of Preeclampsia
Edited by Nidhi Sharma
p. cm.
Print ISBN 978-1-78984-722-2
Online ISBN 978-1-78984-723-9
eBook (PDF) ISBN 978-1-83962-257-1

For EU product safety concerns:
IN TECH d.o.o., Prolaz Marije Krucifikse Kozulić 3, 51000 Rijeka, Croatia, info@intechopen.com or visit our website at intechopen.com.

Meet the editor

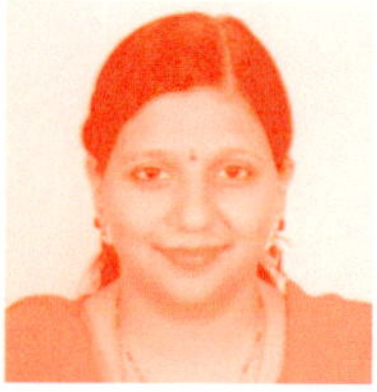

Dr. Nidhi Sharma obtained her MBBS and MS from Banaras Hindu University, Varanasi, India. She is Fellow of the Indian College of Obstetrics and Gynecology, Fellow of assisted reproductive techniques, and Professor of Obstetrics and Gynecology at Saveetha University, India. Dr. Sharma has 60 indexed publications and has authored several chapters in textbooks. She received her PhD degree in Obstetrics and Gynecology from Saveetha University, India, and Diploma in IVF and Reproductive Medicine from UKSH Universitätsklilikum Schleswig-Holstein, Germany. Dr Sharma has been a member of the teaching faculty of MBBS and MS for twelve years.

Contents

Foreword

Prediction of Maternal and Fetal Syndrome of Preeclampsia provides comprehensive information about preeclampsia, including a set of tentative specific prediction markers that can be used to identify different subtypes of the condition, classify pathogenesis, categorize treatment, and identify early signs of complications.

Section 1 deals with etiology of preeclampsia, risk factors, and biomarkers. Section 2 discusses biochemical markers, placental adaptation, autophagy, alteration in erythrocytes, and the association of preeclampsia with gestational diabetes and adolescent pregnancy.

Written by international experts in the field, this volume approaches the topic with an eye toward early detection and treatment.

I congratulate all the authors for their tremendous effort in bringing this book to publication.

N. Hephziabh Kirubamani
M.D, D.G.O, F.R.C.O.G, F.I.C.O.G, PhD, D.Sc.,
Prof. Saveetha Medical College, SIMAT

Preface

Written by international authors and researchers, this book provides a comprehensive overview of preeclampsia and attempts to define biophysical and biochemical markers of the condition.

The first chapter in Section 1 provides an overview of preeclampsia, describing the various subtypes and their clinical features. Since the etiology and pathogenesis isof preeclampsia are segregated and multifactorial, there can beis no single clinical, clinical, biophysical, or biochemical marker that can predict all types of preeclampsia. The second chapter in this section discusses the various clinical, biochemical, and biophysical markers of the subtypes of preeclampsia.

In Section 2, chapters examine preeclampsia in different populations. These subpopulations not only have different clinical risk factors but they also have different symptomatology and biochemical and echocardiography features. Chapters in this section address placental hypoxia, autophagy, impaired lipid peroxidation, oxidative stress, microvasculopathies like diabetes, and subsequent epigenetic and immunogenic modifications.

The chapter on biochemical alterations describes the mediators released by the feto-placental-maternal unit. The chapter on placental adaptation gives a clear insight into the functioning of the placenta. How the placenta copes with diminished blood supply is different from any other tissue of the human body. The chapter on autophagy in the placenta is a new concept of deranged apoptosis and genetic regulations of delayed and reduced apoptotic shedding. Altered zeta potential of red blood cells and endothelial cell dysfunction, though they proceed the clinical manifestation, are a late result of mediators released from placental adaptations to oxidative stress, immunologically damage, hypoxia, and lipid peroxidation.

Gestational diabetes raises the risk of preeclampsia. The epigenetics of preeclampsia are modified due to hyperglycemia in pregnancy. The chapter on diabetes and preeclampsia unravels the mystery of this strong association. The chapter on adolescent pregnancy and preeclampsia emphasizes the immunogenic cause of preeclampsia.

An individualized rational approach to treating preeclampsia in different populations is required. This book is an attempt to sub classify preeclampsia and use these classifications to predict treatment outcomes. Studies conducted in the past have provided significant new insights and these new concepts would not have been possible without the efforts of numerous researchers who continue working on preeclampsia.

Nidhi Sharma
Saveetha University,
Chennai, Tamil Nadu, India

Section 1

Etiopathogenesis and Risk Assessment

Chapter 1

Introductory Chapter: The Multiple Etiologies of Preeclampsia

Nidhi Sharma

Preeclampsia is an "old" disease. "After more than a century of intensive research, preeclampsia and eclampsia remain an enigmatic set of conditions."
Roberts JM, Cooper DW. Pathogenesis and genetics of preeclampsia. Lancet. 2001;357:53e6.

1. Introduction

Preeclampsssia or "gestosis" or "toxemia of pregnancy" is any condition predisposing to eclampsia or convulsions during pregnancy. The word eclampsia is derived from a Greek word *eklampsis* meaning "lightening" or convulsions. Preeclampsia is speculated to be a heterogeneous group of disorders caused by multiple etiologies. Understanding the pathophysiology of this syndrome is important as different etiologies have different pathological mechanisms and different predictive markers. Though the defect could have arisen in the renin-angiotensin system, cardiovascular system, liver enzyme deficiency, coagulation cascade, oxidative stress, or placental bed, the clinical picture is usually oversimplified as the maternal syndrome of hypertension, edema, and proteinuria.

The third world countries will benefit from the provision of adequate antenatal care after these high-risk women are identified. In the developed world, however, the emphasis is on early detection and prevention of preeclampsia.

During pregnancy, the physiology of cardiovascular system, renin-angiotensin system, pancreas changes, different organ reserves are put to test. Understanding preeclampsia requires the understanding of physiology of pregnancy. The blood flow in multiple organs is increased (**Figure 1**). Numerous studies at the embryo-endometrial interphase have also suggested the association of impaired spiral artery remodeling in preeclampsia, but how exactly is the impaired remodeling mediated and what is the pathogenesis of maternal syndrome are still to be elucidated. Some clinical cases of maternal syndrome of preeclampsia also have normal placental histology, so all cases cannot be attributed to a primary placental defect.

Clinical, biochemical, and biophysical markers are used for prediction depending on the etiology of the maternal syndrome of preeclampsia in the pregnancy (**Figure 2a** and **b**). These biomarkers can specifically be used to diagnose the etiology of maternal syndrome as renal dysfunction (kallikrein-creatinine ratio, angiotensin sensitivity test), vascular resistance (uterine artery Doppler), coagulation disorders (platelet volume, fibronectin, prostacyclin, thromboxane), oxidative stress (lipid peroxidase, 8-isoprostane, antioxidants, anticardiolipin antibodies, homocysteine), vascular adaptation (placental growth factor, vascular endothelial growth factor, s-flut, sEng), and placental dysfunction and ischemia (placental CRH, CRH bp, activin, inhibin, hCG).

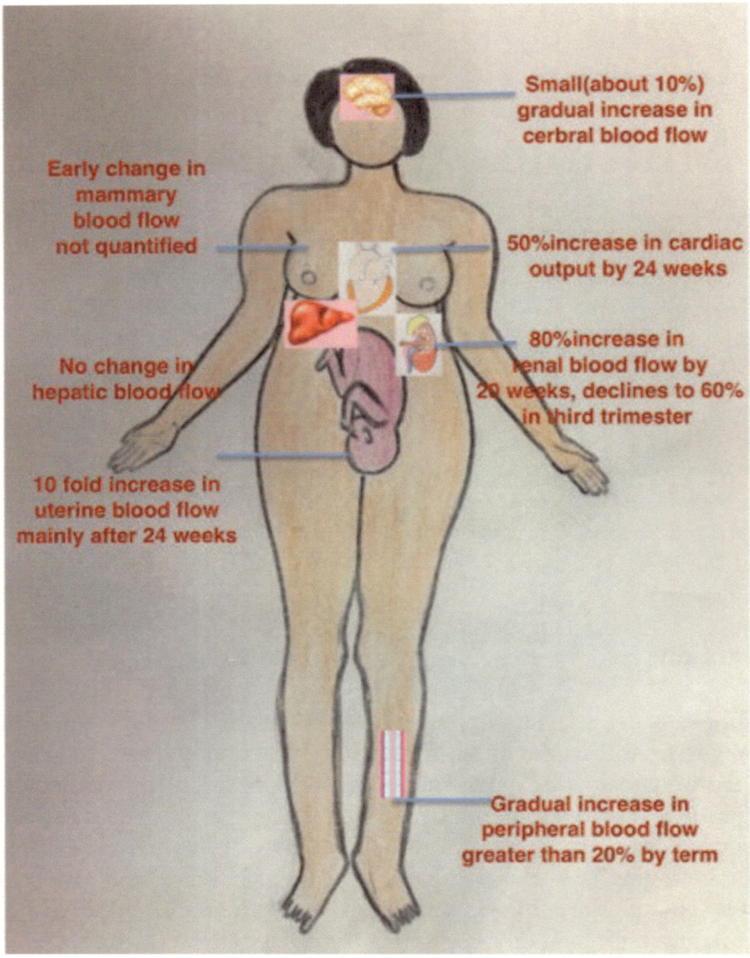

Figure 1.
The distribution of blood flow to maternal organs during pregnancy.

Atypical postpartum preeclampsia has an entirely different pathophysiology; it can be associated with the puerperal defects that prevent the excretion of sodium, puerperal diuresis. It can also be caused by an impaired shift of intravascular fluid into the extravascular compartment (atrial natriuretic peptide in the first week after delivery, natriuresis and inhibition of aldosterone, angiotensin II, vasopressin).

In this chapter the emphasis is on the preclinical pathophysiology of stage 1 of preeclampsia before the development of clinically evident stage 2 of hypertension, edema, and proteinuria.

There are two sides of fetal maternal interface, the maternal and the fetal. At the maternal side, the most important change is the remodeling of the spiral arterioles in the uterine endometrium and myometrium. The spiral arteries supply the intervillous space with blood in which there are floating fetal villi. Decidual veins drain the intervillous space.

At the fetal side, there is the development of fetal villi containing fetal capillaries. The fetal capillaries are covered by mesenchyme and cytotrophoblast. As the cytotrophoblast proliferates, it differentiates into the syncytiotrophoblast that covers the fetal villi. The cytotrophoblast also penetrates into the decidual stroma as interstitial trophoblast and also into maternal spiral arteries as endovascular trophoblast. The changes on both sides of fetomaternal interphase are described vide infra.

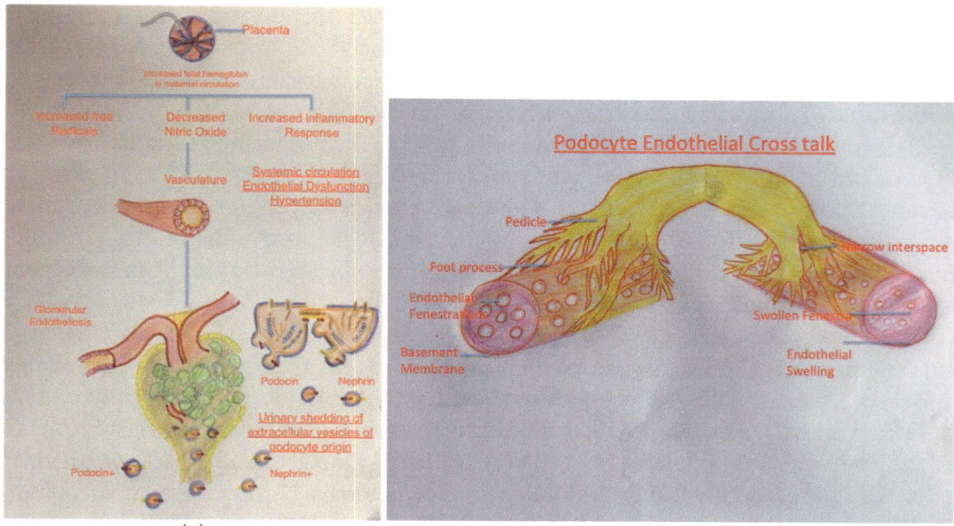

(a) (b)

Figure 2.
(a) Maternal syndrome of edema, hypertension, and proteinuria, and (b) podocyte and endothelial relation in normal pregnancy and preeclampsia.

2. The maternal side of fetoplacental interface

In humans' and primates' placental bed, at the embryo-endometrial interface, the extravillous trophoblastic cells of fetal origin penetrate not only the endometrium but also the subendometrial or junctional zone (JZ) myometrium [1–3]. These fetal origin cells also penetrate the interstitium, block the spiral vessel wall, and finally actually get incorporated into the vessel walls resulting in wide channels ensuring constant slow velocity uninterrupted blood flow to the placental sinuses. The fetal tertiary stem villi bathe in these placental sinuses and are gently sprinkled over by maternal blood [4].

It was emphasized by Brosen et al. [5] that this "physiological transformation" of spiral arterioles at the fetomaternal interphase was a result of the phagocytotic action of rapidly dividing and migrating fetal trophoblast that proliferate on vascular smooth muscles and elastic membranes [6]. Some years later a maternal role in spiral arteriolar remodeling was discovered since a few changes in the maternal vessel wall like dilatation of arterioles, immunosuppression, and rheological changes in the vessel wall and uterine decidua actually happen before the antidromic migration and proliferation of fetal trophoblast along the maternal vessel lumen [7].

The four steps of spiral arteriolar remodeling are explained below [8]. In the first step, there is maternal decidua-associated remodeling independent of the trophoblast. Encircling sheaths of edematous decidual cells around the vessels (Streeter's column) appear as early as postovulatory day 11 [3]. These swollen perivascular cells are usually originated from vascular smooth muscles of spiral arterioles.

At 9 weeks of gestational age of the embryo, the maternal natural killer cells in the uterine decidua synthesize and secrete vascular endothelial growth factor (VEGF), placental growth factor (PLGF), and other angiopoietins [9, 10]. This results in vacuolation and disorganization of endothelial cells in the vascular lumen. In junctional zone or subendometrial myometrium, there are no immune-modified natural killer cells of pregnancy, and the penetrating interstitial trophoblast helps the release of VEGF and angiopoietins [9, 10]. This is concluded because the interstitial trophoblast enters the JZ a little later at 8 weeks.

After this there are actual trophoblastic proliferation and intra-arterial migration. Penetration can happen in the stroma (interstitial trophoblast) or inside the vessels (endovascular trophoblast). The endovascular course only takes place antidromically only in spiral arteries but not in veins (**Figure 3**).

The interstitial trophoblast subsequently fuses to form multinuclear giant cells, but endovascular trophoblast remains mononuclear and with phagocytosis tries to became a part of the vessel wall [11]. Though the multinuclear giant cells appear more evident on histology examination, it is the mononuclear cytotrophoblast that is more phagocytotic, and it proliferates widely the uterine endometrium and JZ myometrium within a short time (**Figure 4**). A large quantity of interstitial trophoblastic cells (basophilic mononuclear cells) proliferate in the extracellular space between the smooth muscles of the JZ myometrium. Trophoblast cells are distributed at the center at 8–14 weeks, and at 16–18 weeks, they are more migrated toward the periphery, thus following an enlarging ringlike pattern of centrifugal migration toward the periphery of the placental bed [12]. It is believed that as the trophoblastic cells fuse to form giant cells, they are gradually losing the ability for phagocytosis. During the transformation of the endometrium to decidua, there is a selective breakdown of extracellular matrix of stroma, and this occurs independent of fetal trophoblastic action.

The interstitial migration and proliferation of trophoblast into the decidua and JZ myometrium (extravascular trophoblast) precede the proliferation of trophoblast spiral arteries (endovascular trophoblast) by several weeks. The first thing the proliferating endovascular mononuclear trophoblast does is to plug the outlets of spiral arterioles at the fetomaternal interface and thus create a low-oxygen environment for the developing embryo. The embryo cannot tolerate a high oxygen tension. After 10 weeks the entire span of the spiral arteries in decidua contains trophoblast reaching even up to the superficial vascular JZ myometrium. Deep invasion of myometrial segments of the spiral arteries happens only after 15 weeks (the second wave of proliferation).

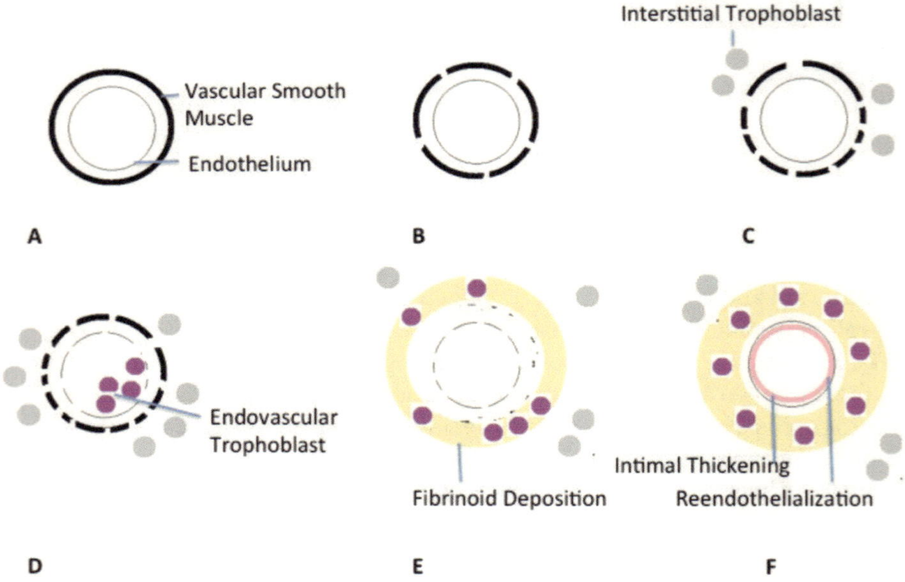

Figure 3.
(A) Unmodified spiral artery showing endothelium and vascular smooth muscle, (B) Decidua associated remodeling with disorganization of vascular smooth muscles, (C) Interstitial Trophoblast migration enhances vascular smooth muscle disorganization, (D) Endovascular Trophoblast temporarily replaces to endothelium, (E) Intramural incorporation of endovascular trophoblast and deposition of fibrinoid, replacing the vascular smooth muscle, (F) Reendothelialisation and intimal thickening.

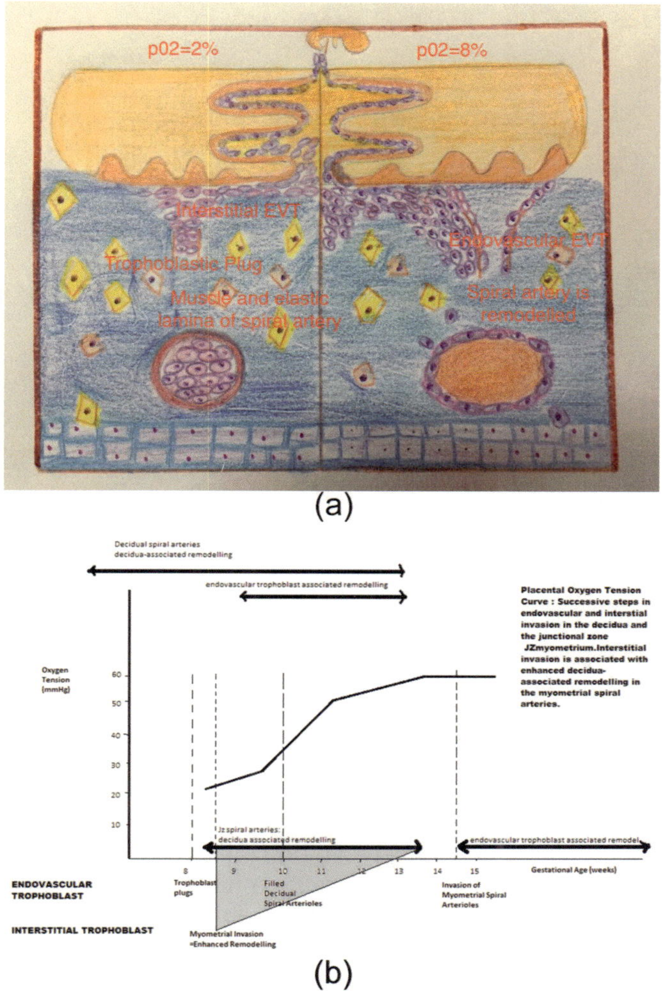

Figure 4.
(a) Placental oxygen tension curve, (b) trophoblastic penetration and placental oxygenation at 7–11 and 12–16 weeks.

The third step is called as trophoblast-induced remodeling when the trophoblast cells actually become a part of the arterial wall. This vascular incorporation happens when the fetal trophoblast actually penetrates the maternal endothelium. Electron micrography studies of maternal decidua have revealed that the trophoblast penetrates between the healthy endothelial cells and crosses the underlying basement membrane. The smooth muscle penetration results in replacement of maternal endothelial cells with trophoblast embedded within a fibroid matrix, probably secreted by the trophoblast itself. The intraluminal trophoblastic cells now incorporated into the vessel wall now assume a spiderlike shape because of increasing accumulation of fibrinoid materials around the cell processes. The intraluminal trophoblast always remains mononuclear or at the most becomes binuclear. This is opposite to the interstitial trophoblast.

The fourth step of re-endothelialization occurs when the maternal vascular lining is repaired by endothelial remnants, which were still present after the intramural invasion. A new endothelial covering may also be derived from circulating endothelial progenitor cells.

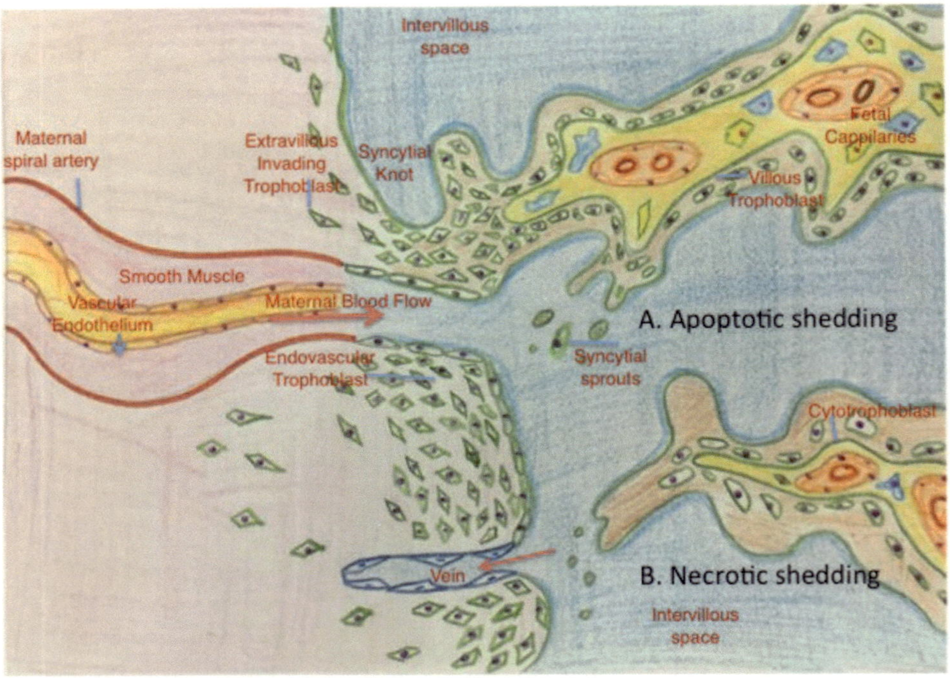

Figure 5.
(a) Syncytial apoptotic shedding in normal pregnancy, (b) trophoblastic penetration and proliferation in preeclampsia.

Investigations of Jauniaux have outlined the different times in gestation at which the decidual spiral arteries and junctional zone spiral arteries get remodeled in decidual association (step 1) and endovascular trophoblast association (step 2). Placental oxygenation increases as gestation advances (**Figure 4a** and **b**). There is no connection between the spiral arteries and the intervillous space at 7 weeks. And they appear at 8 weeks. Even before this communication, the decidual spiral arteries have remodeled (**Figure 5**). At 7–10 weeks, there is first wave of remodeling of decidual spiral arteries and early rise of intervillous flow. The second wave of remodeling, from 15 weeks onward, in which the endovascular trophoblast is observed in the junctional myometrium, is well after the steep rise in placental oxygenation. The decidua-associated spiral remodeling of the myometrium happens at 8–14 weeks, while trophoblastic-associated remodeling of the myometrium happens only after 15 weeks. The early decidua-associated remodeling of the junctional myometrium essentially prepares for the rise in uteroplacental flow, while the subsequent trophoblast-associated remodeling only stabilizes the vessel, and the increased flow is maintained.

2.1 Topology of vascular remodeling

A lateral gradient of diminished invasion has been seen at the periphery of the placental bed as compared to the center of the placental bed. Even in normal pregnancies, the junctional myometrium spiral arteries are remodeled only at the center, and there is an absence of junctional zone myometrial vascular remodeling at the periphery of the placental bed. In preeclampsia the trophoblast-associated remodeling is restricted to the decidual spiral arteries even in the center of the placental bed. One

High risk	Possible explanation	Prediction by	Clinical features
Teenage pregnancy, short interval of pregnancy since menarche, no prior intercourse, and primipaternity	Defective infiltration of decidua by natural killer cells, ligand receptor interaction of leukocyte populations	Maternal history	Maternal syndrome, proteinuria, hypertension, edema
Molar pregnancy	Failed trophoblastic migration and intersignal. Ineffective blocking of spiral vessels and oxidative stress and embryo-endometrial interphase	Early first trimester scan	
Chronic hypertension, high altitude pregnancy, increased maternal age, and diabetes	Impaired apoptosis of hyperplastic arterial smooth muscles of spiral arteries	Maternal history, insulin resistance, glucose intolerance	
Connective tissue disorders, SLE, APLA. Factor 2 and factor 5 Leiden mutations, serpin gene mutations, and protein C and protein S deficiencies	Impaired fibrin deposition by trophoblasts	APLA, ANA, protein essay and genetic screening	
Rh incompatibility, hyperhomocysteinemia	Exaggerated maternal healing tissue response	ABO incompatibility, Rh incompatibility screening	
Vascular resistance	Noncompliant maternal cardiovascular system	Uteroplacental artery flow waveforms, angiotensin II type 1 receptor agonistic antibodies	
Oxidant stress	Lipid peroxidase, 8-isoprostane, antioxidants, hypertriglyceridemia, hemoglobin, iron, transferrin, albumin isoforms	Serum levels, plasma and tissue expression of the long pentraxin 3	
Renal disease	Kallikrein-creatinine	Serum/urine levels	
Coagulation, fibrinolysis system, platelet activation, markers of vascular function	Platelet volume, fibronectin, prostacyclin, thromboxane	Serum levels	
Placental ischemia secondary to any of the above	Placental peptides, CRH, CRH bp, activin, inhibin, HCG	Ratio of angiogenic (placental growth factors, VEGF) and antiangiogenic factors (s-flut and s-endoglin)	

High risk	Possible explanation	Prediction by	Clinical features
Postpartum preeclampsia, inadequate mobilization of liquid from the interstitial and intravascular to extravascular space (6–8 L of the total body water, return of 950 mEq of total body sodium accumulated during pregnancy)	Factors affecting increased urinary sodium excretion between 3 and 5 days after birth (increase of atrial natriuretic peptide in the first week after delivery, natriuresis and inhibition of aldosterone, angiotensin II, vasopressin)	Central venous pressure and pulmonary capillary wedge pressures, colloid osmotic pressure, pulmonary crept, clinical congestive heart failure, cerebral edema	Postpartum convulsions due to posterior reversible encephalopathy syndrome—vasogenic edema in posterior brain due to lack of sympathetic modulation

Table 1.
Possible prediction of various subtypes of preeclampsia.

study demonstrated that even decidual segments might show incomplete remodeling. It is imperative that the placental bed biopsy should be taken from an adequately central space and not lateral. There are less interstitial giant cells in the myometrium and more stacked endometrial glands pushed by the placenta at the periphery of the placental bed.

2.2 Failure of remodeling

2.2.1 Failure of step 1: decidua-associated remodeling is defective

Late luteal phase secretory endometrium decidualization is associated with infiltration of natural killer cells, which are now considered to be major effector cells at trophoblast-uterine interphase interactions. It has also been postulated that repeated cycles of menstrual shedding of decidualizing endometrium may act as preconditioning for successful implantation and deep placentation [13]. This might explain the increased risk of preeclampsia in teenage pregnancy, short interval of pregnancy since menarche, and primipaternity. This may also explain the lowered risk of preeclampsia in women who have intercourse earlier with partner who fathers the current pregnancy. Recent research also suggests that natural killer cells' associated defects of implantation are due to disturbed ligand receptor interphase. Uterine natural killer cells are absent in the JZ myometrium, but their angiogenic action is mediated by interstitial trophoblast.

2.2.2 Failure of step 2: failed trophoblastic migration

An impaired rise in blood flow, as a result of improper decidualization and improper angiogenesis, leads to a failed integrin shift and a failure of trophoblast to acquire an endothelial phenotype. Disturbed HLA-G expression by trophoblast has also been postulated. This might explain preeclampsia seen in association with molar pregnancy.

2.2.3 Failure of step 3: trophoblast-associated remodeling is defective

Impaired intramural incorporation of endovascular trophoblast and lack of fibrin deposition can be caused by impaired secretion of proteinases. This may be because of improper trophoblast signaling. This might explain the increased risk preeclampsia in connective tissue disorders, SLE, and APLA. The defective laying down of fibrin may explain the preeclampsia in cases of thrombophilia disorders like factor 2 and factor 5 Leiden mutations, serpin gene mutations, and protein C and protein S deficiencies. This might also explain the association of preeclampsia with placenta accreta and increta where the Nitabuch's layer is absent. Chronic hypertension, renal disease, increased maternal age, and diabetes may lead to hyperplasia of smooth muscles of spiral arterial media; this may lead to impaired maintenance of elastin and vascular smooth muscles [14, 15]. When these conditions are present subclinically before pregnancy, the preexisting Tunica media hyperplasia might interfere with trophoblast-induced apoptosis of elastic smooth muscles.

2.2.4 Failure of step 4: increased maternal inflammatory response

Trophoblast proliferation and apoptosis of maternal intra-arterial smooth muscles invariable incites maternal tissue repair mechanisms, it is easy to understand that if maternal inflammation is marked the proliferating trophoblast may be destroyed by lipophages resulting in "acute atherosis lesions" in the placental bed [16]. This might explain the occurrence of preeclampsia in Rh-incompatible pregnancies and hyperhomocysteinemia (**Table 1**).

3. The fetal side of fetoplacental interface

Syncytial sprouts arise from the syncytiotrophoblast that covers the cytotrophoblast around the fetal stem villi. In early pregnancy large aggregates of trophoblastic cells proliferate and extend into the intervillous space forming drumstick-like syncytial structures. Syncytial sprouts are multinucleated and have large ovoid nuclei with very little heterochromatin. There are a large number of ribosomes with abundant rough endoplasmic reticulum. Larger nuclei are present in the sprouts as compared to other parts of syncytiotrophoblast. True sprouts are produced from the mesenchyme villi and immature intermediate villi (**Figure 5**). There are continuous differentiation and proliferation of cytotrophoblast into syncytiotrophoblast into sprouts. This can be (a) sprout-like apoptotic shedding, (b) knots or Tenny-Parker changes, (c) wavelike apoptotic shedding, (d) arrested apoptotic shedding, (e) aponecrotic shedding, and (e) necrotic shedding.

3.1 Sprout-like apoptotic shedding

This is a normal phenomenon in which villous trophoblast proliferates and differentiates into cytotrophoblast. The cytotrophoblast fuses with the overlying syncytiotrophoblast, and finally the old and aging material is packaged into apoptotic syncytial sprouts and released into the maternal circulation. If apoptotic shedding is blocked, the number of nuclei in the syncytium increases. Since it is a membrane-sealed apoptotic material, it does not induce an inflammatory response. In the maternal lung, the syncytial sprouts get trapped and are phagocytosized by lung macrophages without inflammatory reaction. Approximately 3 g of apoptotically shed trophoblast is destroyed in the lungs daily. This is the balance of 3.6 g of cytotrophoblast that is converted to syncytiotrophoblast each day and 0.6 g that is retained in the syncytium [17, 18].

3.2 Tenny-Parker changes or syncytial knots

The terms syncytial sprouts and syncytial knots are different. True syncytial sprouts happen in first half of pregnancy when they represent early stages of large euchromatic nucleus. Tenny-Parker changes also called as syncytial knots are bridges between the neighboring villi that look like drumstick or mushroomlike projections containing normally structured nuclei. These are artifacts caused by tangential sectioning of highly branched fetal villi.

3.3 Wavelike apoptotic shedding

In cases of placentas of fetal growth restricted with absent diastolic flow, there is a large decrease in the number of cytotrophoblastic cells, and the thickness of syncytiotrophoblast is also less [19]. The nuclei in syncytiotrophoblast accumulate like a ring around the vertical axis of villi. The underlying pathology is yet to be identified [17, 18].

3.4 Arrested apoptotic shedding

Apoptotic syncytial nuclei accumulate in knot-like structures but do not get extruded into the intervillous space. This is also seen in the cases of fetal growth restriction with absent diastolic flow. At some places the sites with nuclei are even larger than the cross section of villi from which they arise. It is seen that a large number of these giant knots form all over the placenta. In these cases the apoptotic cleavage of syncytial cytoskeleton may be defective [17, 18].

3.5 Aponecrotic shedding

Aponecrosis is a term used when signs of apoptotic trophoblast turnover and shedding are associated with signs of syncytial necrosis. Apoptosis continues with damaged plasma membranes, water influx and secondary hydropic changes of cellular structures, and release of cytoplasmic contents. This process is also called as secondary necrosis. Since apoptosis is a programmed cell death depending on cell energy, lack of cell energy reserves could be the cause of aponecrosis. These villous explants contain cell-free DNA, cell-free actin, and membrane-wrapped nuclei. In some studies in preeclampsia, the villous explants that had the packaged nuclei showed early signs of chromatin condensation, but the cytoplasm was edematous and plasma membrane had local defects.

3.6 Necrotic shedding

In pure necrotic shedding, the villous explants contain edematous nuclei in a hydropic cytoplasm with membrane defects. Placentas from severe preeclampsia and severe Rh incompatibility have shown features of necrotic shedding. The complete absence of chromatin condensation showed that the apoptotic pathway was blocked by inhibitory proteins and never restarted. In an experiment on pregnant guinea pigs, complete blockage of energy metabolism of trophoblast was done by monoiodine acetate or sodium fluoride (inhibitors of glycolysis). Continuous release of necrotic villous explants leads to the features of pre-eclampsia [17, 18].

If cytotrophoblast keeps growing and accumulating as syncytiotrophoblast and does not shed, it will lead to intrasyncytial accumulation of old and aged trophoblastic components which finally necrose. Cytoplasmic blebbing of syncytium with nuclear and cytoplasmic edema is a hallmark feature of necrotic shedding. Though there are phenotypic similarities among different types of villous explants, there are differences in modes of nuclear chromatin aggregation, nuclear or cytosolic edema. Cracks in the plasma membrane help to differentiate between physiological apoptotic shedding and pathological necrotic shedding.

4. Placenta as a casualty and not the cause

4.1 Liver pathology as a cause of preeclampsia

Preeclampsia is associated with three unique liver lesions described as liver lesions of preeclampsia, HELLP syndrome, and acute fatty liver of pregnancy. HELLP syndrome has classical periportal or focal parenchymal liver necrosis. There is thrombotic microangiopathy with resulting hemolysis and liver damage. Few cases of HELLP are associated with defects in beta-oxidation of fatty acids. There is microangiopathic hemolytic anemia with schistocytes, thrombocytopenia, and elevated levels of ALT/AST/LDH/bilirubin. HELLP may even develop postpartum, so the placenta is an unlikely cause of HELLP syndrome (**Figure 6**).

Acute fatty liver of pregnancy is due to defective oxidation of beta fatty acids. There is mitochondrial deficiency of long-chain 3-hydroxyacyl coenzyme A dehydrogenase in fetus. This leads to accumulation of 3-hydroxyacyl metabolites that are toxic to the liver. Half of the pregnancies with acute fatty liver of pregnancy develop preeclampsia (**Figure 7**).

4.2 Renin-angiotensin system as a cause of preeclampsia

The renin-angiotensin system (RAS) recognizes pregnancy very early. In the luteal phase of menstrual cycle, the RAS is activated under the influence of progesterone, and if pregnancy occurs, this RAS activation is maintained. This activation of RAS may be caused by progesterone that is natriuretic or it could be the "perceived under filling" of circulation by macula densa in early pregnancy. Juxtaglomerular apparatus synthesizes and releases renin, an aspartyl protease. Estrogen simultaneously binds to the promoter region of alpha-2 globulin angiotensinogen (AOGEN) and leads to the synthesis of angiotensinogen. Plasma

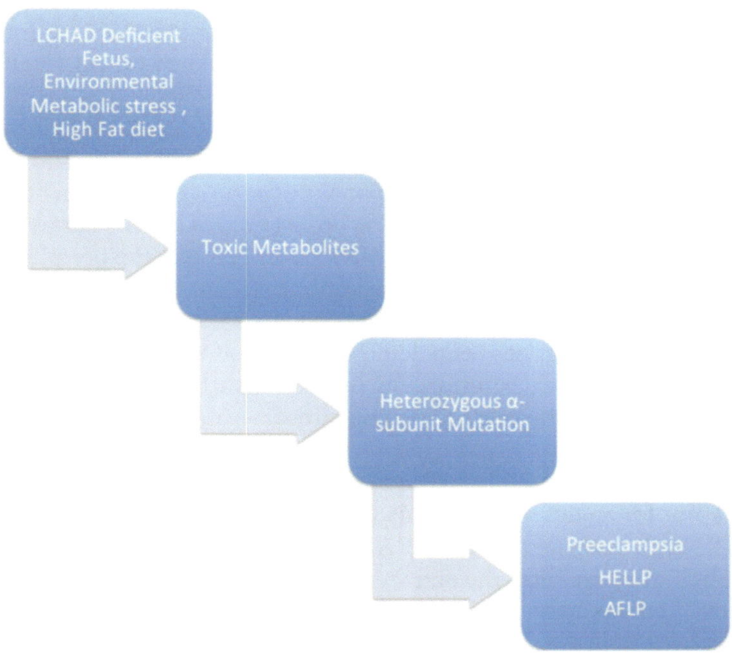

Figure 6.
Pathogenesis of preeclampsia in LACHD deficient fetus.

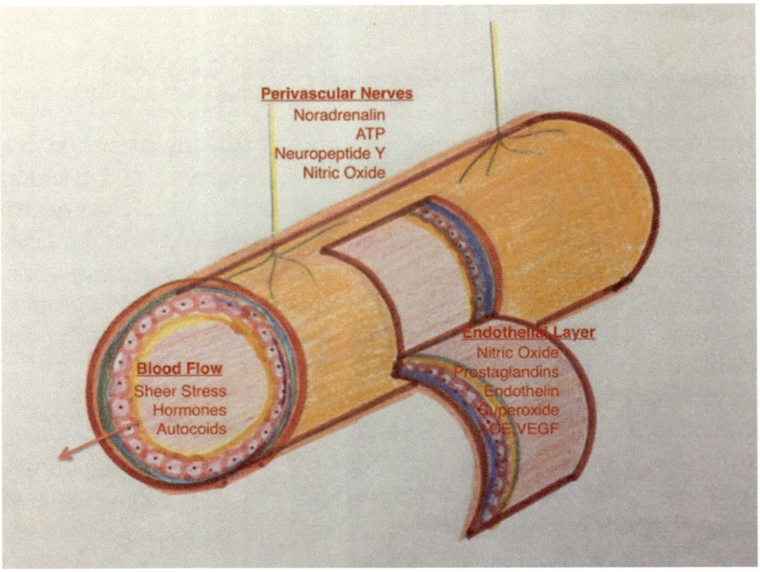

Figure 7.
Pathogenesis of preeclampsia in a nonresilient cardiovascular system. The autonomic nervous system, intrinsic smooth muscle reflexes, and the endothelium influence vascular tone.

angiotensin II (AGII) rises and leads to the synthesis and release of aldosterone from the zona glomerulosa in the adrenal cortex. The pregnant women do not develop hypertension from the presser effects of AGII due to the downregulation of ATR1 receptors. The vessel responsive to adrenal cortisol is usually unaltered in pregnancy [20, 21].

Angiotensin II is very peculiar because its action depends on which of its two receptors it is acting. When AGII binds with AGI receptors, it causes vasoconstriction, but when it binds to AGII receptors, it causes vasodilation. If angiotensin I receptors are downregulated during pregnancy or by angiotensin receptor blockers like telmisartan or if angiotensin II receptors are upregulated during fetal life, it is a vasodilator.

Villous syncytiotrophoblast has high density of angiotensinase A (aminopeptidase A) which converts angiotensin II to angiotensin III [22, 23]. The increase in this angiotensinase activity is also responsible for downregulation of ATR1 receptors in normal pregnancy [24]. It was observed that during cesarean section in normal pregnancy, the uterine venous AGII is lower than the peripheral venous AGII. In preeclampsia pregnancy, uterine venous AGII are higher than peripheral AGII level [25].

In prospective studies it has been demonstrated that aminopeptidase A levels were high before the clinical syndrome of preeclampsia but levels were lower after preeclampsia clinically developed [24]. The initial rise in trophoblastic aminopeptidase could be an initial homeostatic response protecting placenta from the harmful effects of locally generated AGII.

The receptor for angiotensin IV is also called as insulin-regulated aminopeptidase (IRAP). High concentrations of IRAP are present on human placenta [26]. In the second half of pregnancy, the extracellular domain of this receptor is shed off. Angiotensin IV acts as an endogenous inhibitor of angiotensin-converting enzyme. It stimulates both RNA and DNA synthesis in endothelial cells and proliferation of endothelial cells. It can also increase the levels of plasminogen activator inhibitor mRNA. It is a vasodilator at least in cerebral vessels. These features are important because angiotensin IV can be involved in local apoptosis and remodeling.

4.3 Noncompliant cardiovascular system as a cause of preeclampsia

In preeclampsia there may be an impaired vasodilator response to endothelium-dependent agonists such as acetylcholine and bradykinin (**Figure 7**). Various adaptive mechanisms are employed at the fetomaternal interphase, and subsequently after 20 weeks, a clinically evident maternal syndrome of hypertension, edema, and proteinuria develops. The development of second stage of late vascular dysfunction can also happen independent of first stage. The uterine artery Doppler waveform becomes transformed into a high flow with low resistance at 22–24 weeks in normal gestation. However, in preeclampsia there is a latent preclinical stage with impaired intravascular volume expansion, hyperdynamic circulation, and a decreased cardiac output as clinical disease develops. This decreased cardiac output leads to renal and uteroplacental insufficiency. There may also be leaky capillaries leading to pulmonary and cerebral edema. Severe and early-onset preeclampsia has abnormal uterine artery waveform in preclinical stage and hypertension in clinical stage. Abnormal Doppler of uterine artery may be considered as a local noninvasive imaging of a more generalized systemic vasculopathy. This may mediate further cardiovascular risks. Women with preeclampsia are also two and a half times likely to die from ischemic heart disease in later life [27–29]. Several studies have been conducted showing preeclampsia association with the high pulsatility index of uterine artery.

Raised uterine artery impedance is a marker of early endothelial dysfunction. It is associated with increased aortic pulse wave velocity and augmentation index in the first trimester of pregnancy that is the marker of future cardiovascular risk [30–32]. Increased homocysteine levels have also been implicated in both cardiovascular risks and preeclampsia [33].

5. Conclusion

Preeclampsia is a heterogeneous disease. The late-onset preeclampsia at or near term has low fetal and maternal morbidity. But the early-onset preeclampsia (1%) of all preeclampsia has significant risks. Prediction of risks and identification of subclinical disease are mandatory. The majority of at-risk groups in multigravida are chronic hypertension, pregestational and gestational diabetes, age, and multiple fetuses, whereas in primigravida only 14% have these risks. If there is preeclampsia in a multigravida, a nonplacental cause should be definitely considered. This suggests that there are multiple underlying etiologies of different clinical presentations. **Table 1** summarizes the likely etiopathogenesis in different clinical scenarios. Postpartum eclampsia can be predicted and monitored with central venous pressure and pulmonary capillary wedge pressure [34–36]. The maternal syndrome (proteinuria, edema, and hypertension) also has differences in time of onset, severity, and organ system involvement as highlighted in several studies [37–39]. There is a rising interest in galectin molecules for prediction of these subtypes (**Figure 8**). These clinical subpopulations need to be identified and preeclampsia predicted with rigorous definition of different biomarkers of different clinical phenotypes [40–44]. The future endeavors should be to identify subclinical disease in various clinical phenotypes with these potential biomarkers in prospective longitudinal studies.

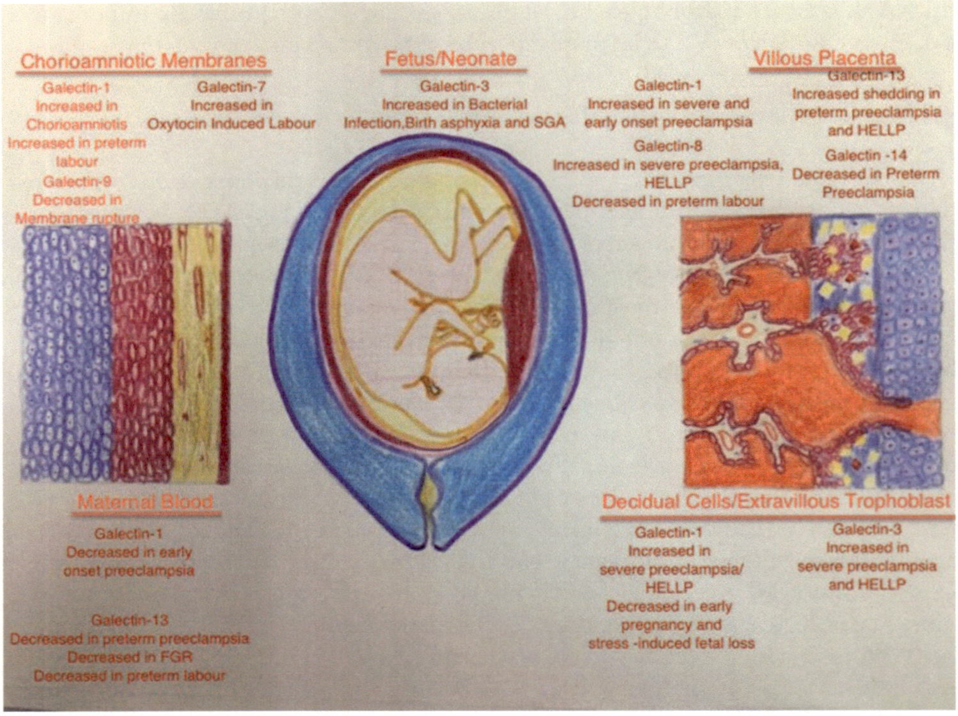

Figure 8.
Galectin subtypes and prediction of preeclampsia.

Author details

Nidhi Sharma
Saveetha University, Chennai, Tamil Nadu, India

*Address all correspondence to: drbonuramkumar@yahoo.co.in

References

[1] Hamilton WJ, Boyd JD. Development of the human placenta in the first three months of gestation. Journal of Anatomy. 1960;**94**:297-328

[2] Hamilton WJ, Boyd JD. Trophoblast in human placental arteries. Nature. 1966;**212**:906-908

[3] Harris JWS, Ramsey EM. The morphology of human uteroplacental vasculature. Contributions to Embryology. 1966;**38**:43-58

[4] Kaufmann P, Black S, Huppertz B. Endovascular trophoblast invasion: Implications for the pathogeneses of intrauterine growth retardation and preeclampsia. Biology of Reproduction. 2003;**69**:1-7

[5] Brosens I, Robertson WB, Dixon HG. The physiological response of the vessels of placental bed to normal pregnancy. The Journal of Pathology and Bacteriology. 1967;**93**:569-579

[6] Pijenborg R, Vercruysse L, Hanssens M. The uterine spiral arteries in human pregnancy: Facts and controversies. Placenta. 1998;**19**:241-252

[7] Craven CM, Morgan T, Ward K. Decidual spiral artery remodeling begins before cellular interaction with cytotrophoblast. Placenta. 1998;**19**:241-252

[8] Li XF, Charnock-Jones DS, Zhang E, Hiby S, Malik S, Day K, et al. Angiogenic growth factor messenger ribonucleic acids in uterine natural killer cells. The Journal of Clinical Endocrinology and Metabolism. 2001;**86**:1823-1834. PubMed PMID: 11297624

[9] Brosens IA. Uteroplacental Vascular Pathology. European Journal of Obstetrics, Gynecology, and Reproductive Biology. 1975;**5**:47-65. Discussion

[10] Pijenborg R, Bland JM, Robertson WB, Brosens I. Uteroplacental arterial changes related to interstitial trophoblast migration in early human pregnancy. 1983;**4**:397-414

[11] Bulmer JN, Lash GE. Human uterine natural killer cells: A reappraisal. Molecular Immunology. 2005;**42**:511-521

[12] Schiessl B, Innes BA, Bulmer JN. Localization of angiogenic growth factors and their receptors in the human placental bed throughout normal human pregnancy. Placenta. 2009;**30**:79-87

[13] Brosens JJ, Parker MG, McIndoe A, Pijnenborg R, Brosens IA. A role for menstruation in preconditioning the uterus for successful pregnancy. American Journal of Obstetrics and Gynecology. June 2009;**200**(6):615. e1-5

[14] Sheppard BL, Bonnar J. An ultrastructural study of utero-placental spiral arteries in hypertensive and normotensive pregnancy and fetal growth retardation. bjog: An International Journal of Obstetrics & Gynaecology. 1981;**88**:695-705. DOI: 10.1111/j.1471-0528.1981.tb01268.x

[15] Robertson WB, Khong TY, Brosens I. The placental bed biopsy: Review from three European centers. American journal of obstetrics and gynaecolgy. Vol. 159:401

[16] Hanssens M, Pijnenborg R, Keire MJNC. Renin-like immunoreactivity in uterus and placenta from normotensive and hypertensive pregnancies. European Journal of Obstetrics, Gynecology, and Reproductive Biology. 1998;**81**:177-184

[17] Pathology of the Human Placenta. 4th Edn. By Kurt Benirschke and Peter Kaufmann. New York: Springer-Verlag, 2000

[18] Kaufmann P, Black S, Huppertz B. Endovascular trophoblast invasion: Implications for the pathogenesis of intrauterine growth retardation and preeclampsia. Biology of Reproduction. 2003;**69**(1):1-7. Epub 2003 Mar 5. Review. PubMed PMID: 12620937

[19] Todros T, Sciarrone A, Piccoli E, Guiot C, Kaufman P, Kingdom J. Umbilical Doppler waveform and placental angiogenesis in pregnancy complicated by fetal growth restriction. Obstetrics and Gynecology. April 1999;**93**:499-503

[20] Baker P, Broughton Pipkin F. AII receptor number and screening for PIH. Clinical and Experimental Pharmacology & Physiology. 1993;**20**(12):809-810. PubMed PMID: 8306522

[21] Skinner SL, Mccubbin JW, Page IH. Renal baroceptor control of renin secretion. Science. 1963;**141**(3583):814-816. PubMed PMID: 14045137

[22] Ino K, Uehara C, Kikkawa F, Kajiyama H, Shibata K, Suzuki T, et al. Enhancement of aminopeptidase A expression during angiotensin II-induced choriocarcinoma cell proliferation through AT1 receptor involving protein kinase C- and mitogen-activated protein kinase-dependent signaling pathway. The Journal of Clinical Endocrinology and Metabolism. 2003;**88**(8):3973-3982. PubMed PMID: 12915695

[23] Johnson AR, Skidgel RA, Gafford JT, Erdös EG. Enzymes in placental microvilli: Angiotensin I converting enzyme, angiotensinase A, carboxypeptidase, and neutral endopeptidase ("enkephalinase"). Peptides. 1984;**5**(4):789-796. PubMed PMID:6093076

[24] Mizutani S, Tomoda Y. Effects of placental proteases on maternal and fetal blood pressure in normal pregnancy and preeclampsia. American Journal of Hypertension. 1996;**9**(6):591-597. Review. PubMed PMID: 8783784

[25] Broughton Pipkin F, Baker PN. Angiotensin II has depressor effects in pregnant and nonpregnant women. Hypertension. 1997;**30**:1247-1252

[26] Albiston AL, Mc Dowall SG, Matasacos D, et al. Evidence that angiotensin IV (AT4) receptor is enzyme insulin regulated aminopeptidase. The Journal of Biological Chemistry. 2001;**276**(48):623-626

[27] Rich Edwards JW, Fraser A, Lawler DA, Catov JM. Pregnancy characteristics and women's future cardiovascular health: An underused opportunity to improve women's health? Epidemiologic Reviews. 2014;**36**:57-70

[28] Fraser A, Nelson SM, Macdonald-Wallis C. Associations of pregnancy complications with calculated cardiovascular risk and cardiovascular risk factors in middle age: The Avon longitudinal study of parents and children. Circulation. 2012;**125**:1367-1380

[29] Brown MC, Best K, Pearce MS, Waugh J, Robson SC, Bell R. Cardiovascular disease risk in women with preeclampsia: Systematic review and meta-analysis. European Journal of Epidemiology. 2013;**28**:1-19

[30] Everett TR, Mahendru AA, McEniery CM, Wilkinson IB, Lees CC. Raised uterine artery impedance is associated with increased arterial stiffness in the late second trimester. Placenta. 2012;**33**:572-577. DOI: 10.1016/j.placenta.2012.04.001. Epub 2012 Apr 24. PMID: 22538229

[31] Savvidou MD, Kaihura C, Anderson JM, Nicolaides KH. Maternal arterial stiffness in women who subsequently develop pre-eclampsia. PLoS One. 2011;**6**:e18703

[32] Macedo ML, Luminoso D, Savvidou MD, McEniery CM, Nicolaides KH. Maternal wave reflections and arterial stiffness in normal pregnancy as assessed by applanation tonometry. Hypertension. 2008;**51**:1047-1051

[33] Yu CKH, Lakasing L, Papageorghiou AT, Spencer K, Nicolaides KH. Uterine artery Doppler and mid-trimester maternal plasma homocysteine in subsequent pre-eclampsia. The Journal of Maternal-Fetal and Neonatal Medicine. **16**:2134-2139

[34] Sanctos M. Evolução dos níveis pressóricos no puerpério em mulheres com pré-eclâmpsia grave atendidas em um hospital terciário: Estudo de coorte [dissertação]. Recife: Instituto de Medicina Integral Professor Fernando Figueira-IMIP; 2004

[35] Pearson JF. Fluid balance in severe preeclampsia. British Journal of Hospital Medicine. 1992;**48**:47-45

[36] Magee Laura, von Dadelszen Peter. Prevention and treatment of postpartum hypertension. Cochrane Database of Systematic Reviews. 30 April 2013:4CD004351. DOI: 10.1002/14651858.CD004351.pub3

[37] Myatt L, Miodovnik M. Prediction of preeclampsia. Seminars in Perinatology. 1999;**23**(1):45-57

[38] Roberts JM, Hubel CA. The two stage model of preeclampsia: Variations on the theme. Placenta. 2009;**30** (Suppl A):S32-S37. DOI: 10.1016/j.placenta.2008.11.009

[39] Roberts J. Pre-eclampsia a two-stage disorder: What is the linkage? Are there directed fetal/placental signals? In: Lyall F, Belfort MA, editors. Pre-eclampsia: Etiology and Clinical Practice. New York: Cambridge University Press; 2007. pp. 183-194

[40] Shibata E, Rajakumar A, Powers RW, Larkin RW, Gilmour C, Bodnar LM, et al. Soluble fms-like tyrosine kinase 1 is increased in preeclampsia but not in normotensive pregnancies with small-for-gestational-age neonates: Relationship to circulating placental growth factor. The Journal of Clinical Endocrinology and Metabolism. 2005;**90**:4895-4903

[41] Walther T, Wallukat G, Jank A, Bartel S, Schultheiss HP, Faber R, et al. Angiotensin II type 1 receptor agonistic antibodies reflect fundamental alterations in the uteroplacental vasculature. Hypertension. 2005;**46**:1275-1279

[42] Vatten LJ, Eskild A, Nilsen TIL, Jeansson S, Jenum PA, Staff AC. Changes in circulating level of angiogenic factors from the first to second trimester as predictors of preeclampsia. American Journal of Obstetrics and Gynecology. 2007;**196**:239.e1-239.e6

[43] Rovere-Querini P, Antonacci S, Dell'Antonio G, Angeli A, Almirante G, Cin ED, et al. Plasma and tissue expression of the long pentraxin 3 during normal pregnancy and preeclampsia. Obstetrics & Gynecology. 2006;**108**:148-155

[44] Ong CY, Liao AW, Spencer K, Munim S, Nicolaides KH. First trimester maternal serum free beta human chorionic gonadotrophin and pregnancy associated plasma protein A as predictors of pregnancy complications. BJOG: An International Journal of Obstetrics & Gynaecology. 2000;**107**:1265-1270

Chapter 2

Risk Factor and Biomarker of Preeclampsia

Makmur Sitepu and Jusuf Rachmadsyah

Abstract

Preeclampsia is a multisystem progressive disorder characterized by new onset of hypertension and proteinuria or hypertension and significant end-organ dysfunction with or without proteinuria after 20 weeks of pregnancy. Recently, it has been shown that early preeclampsia is associated with abnormalities in oxygen sensing since early preeclampsia; the placenta is unable to regulate hypoxia-inducible factor 1- (HIF1-) alpha levels. The risk factors that are involved in the development of preeclampsia are also the symptoms of the metabolic syndrome and glucose metabolism disorders such as diabetes mellitus as well as insulin resistance, increased body mass index (>35 kg/m^2), and elevated diastolic blood pressure > 80 mm Hg. Further risk factors are positive family history of preeclampsia, multiple pregnancy, pregnant women over 40 years, preexisting renal disease, and clotting disorders. All biophysical and biochemical markers are shown to be used for prediction of preeclampsia. Meanwhile, it has been obvious that a single examined marker might not have the conclusion to accurately predict subsequent preeclamptic risk. Consequently, it seems to be convincing to apply history, biophysical, and several biochemical parameters to conclude the best possible detection rate.

Keywords: preeclampsia, maternal risk factors, biophysical, several biochemical parameters

1. Introduction

Preeclampsia is a multisystem progressive disorder characterized by the new onset of hypertension and proteinuria or hypertension and significant end-organ dysfunction with or without proteinuria, in the last half of pregnancy or postpartum. The genesis of the disease is laid down in early pregnancy and is characterized anatomically by abnormal remodeling of the maternal spiral arteries at the placental site.

2–The prevalence of pregnant women affected by preeclampsia (PE) [1] is 7%, commonly occurs in the second half of pregnancy and is basically identified by the existing symptoms of hypertension and proteinuria. HELLP syndrome (hemolysis, elevated liver enzymes, and low platelet count) may develop among 5–8% of these women. Preeclampsia is one of the major triggers of maternal and fetal death worldwide and a common cause of premature labor. Women with preeclamptic history are at high risk for cardiovascular diseases later in life [2]. Lowering morbidity and mortality resulting from this disease of lifestyle changes, and its preventive actions should be the main objective. The preventive treatment for those with the preeclamptic high risk has the potential to be a predictive tool also for anticipating other health disorders with serious consequences for the mothers, their offsprings, and health-care systems themselves.

2. Pathogenesis

The placenta applies a significant factor in the pathogenesis of preeclampsia because the symptoms of PE can happen in molar pregnancy, which lacks a fetus, and the disease disappears once the placenta is delivered.

Uteroplacental vascular insufficiency triggers fetus malnutrition and inadequate oxygen and nutrients. It is then identified clearly that the impact of such undernutrition condition seemingly causes coronary heart disease and hypertension in the future life [3–5]. It is easily noticed that the human placenta is only a temporary organ, but its effect on the fetus is protecting life. The correct function of the placenta necessitates the correct differentiation of the trophectoderm to set up a nutrition link between the embryo and mother [6]. In spite of numerous years of research, a holistic comprehension molecular pathogenesis of preeclampsia remains unidentified.

The present study of pathogenesis of preeclampsia carried out by Christopher Redman and Ian Sergent is assumed to happen in two-phase series of unsuitable placental condition in the first and at the beginning of the second trimester, and it badly influences the rest of the pregnancy period [7, 8]. Anatomically, placental diagnosis uncovers that the most affected part of this illness is basal plate in which the cytotrophoblast (CBT) exists [9]. In preeclamptic condition, both interstitial CTB and endovascular invasion are not deep, and consequently, it triggers impaired vascular remodeling of the spiral arteries [10]. The next phase of preeclampsia is assumed maternity-related reactions to abnormal placentation as a consequence of endothelial dysfunction and an imbalance in circulating angiogenic/vasculogenic factors such as soluble vascular endothelial growth factor receptor-1 (VEGFR-1, sFlt-1), placental growth factor (PlGF), and the changing complete growth of factor-beta receptor endoglin (CD105) [9, 11, 12] (**Figure 1**).

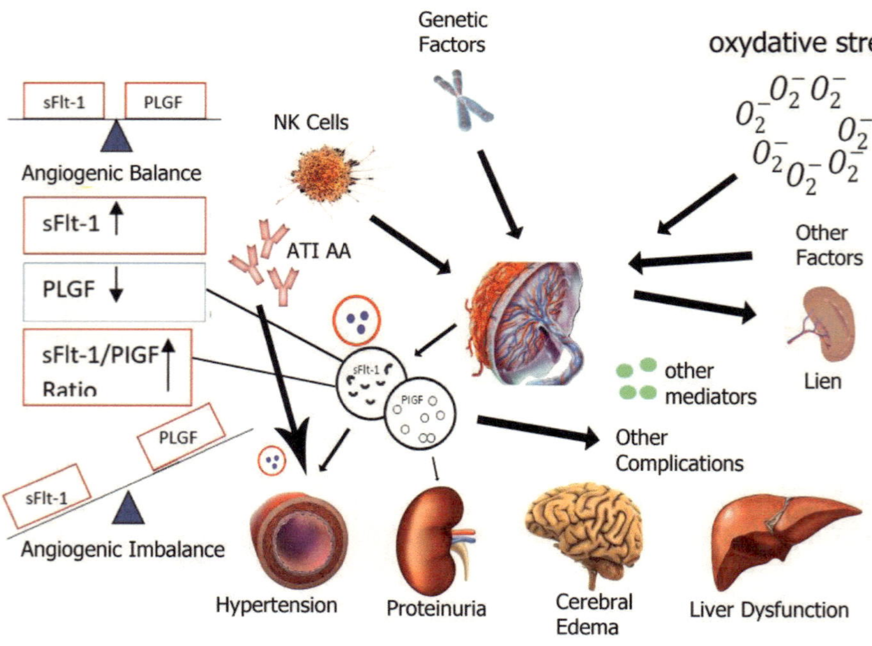

Figure 1.
In normal pregnancies, sFlt-1 and PIGF are in physiological angiogenic balance. Various factors and mediators influence the trophoblast invasion and placentation and in case of preeclampsia cause excessive production and liberation of sFlt-1 levels result in an unphysiological increase of the sFlt-1/PIGF ratio (angiogenic imbalance). Measurement of sFlt-1/PIGF ratio helps to identify women with preeclampsia and those who are likely to develop preeclampsia. ATI AA, angiotensin-converting enzyme autoantibodies. NK cells, natural killer cells.

2.1 New insights of molecule

There is substantial fact that a nonphysiological hypoxic environment subsequently in pregnancy could create such decontrol of angiogenic factors at the motherly embryonic connection. Lately, it has been indicated that the early preeclampsia is linked to anomalies regarding O_2 sensing since preliminary preeclamptic placentas failed to control hypoxia-inducible factor 1- (HIF1-) alpha levels [13]. Incessant vulnerability in nonphysiological O_2 levels in preeclampsia lowers vascular endothelial growth factor (VEGF), whereas sFlt-1 is really responsive. It is clearly accepted that produced sFlt-1 tied to VEGF and PlGF with huge similarity and consequently lowers their ability to link to their receptors [14]. The transformations act like an antiangiogenic treatment indicated in medical tests influencing similar medical symptoms such as angiogenesis dysfunction especially in vessels maturity, hypertension, proteinuria, and edema [14, 15]. Verlohren et al. [16] stated that the sFlt-1/PlGF ratio is essential to recognize females at risk for delivery and is a convincing tool to differentiate between different types of pregnancy-related hypertensive illnesses. Females are classified preeclamptic, at gestational age <34 weeks; the circulating sFlt-1/PlGF ratio predicts adverse outcomes occurring within 2 weeks [17, 18]. However, the mechanisms by which placenta-derived sFlt-1 gains access to the maternal circulation remain unclear. Rajakumar et al. [19] report that the sFlt-1 protein is highly enriched in syncytial knots which is easily detach from the syncytiotrophoblast—a finding which is increased in preeclampsia. These multinucleated aggregates are metabolically active and are capable of de novo synthesis and may thus contribute to the maternal vascular injury in PE [19].

Moreover we revealed a deregulated expression of another molecule found in the bulk of changed molecules in PE: the matricellular CCN3 protein which lead to an imbalance in proliferation and migration of human trophoblast cells and could contribute to the shallow invasion of trophoblast cells into the decidual compartment and spiral arteries observed in preeclampsia [20–23]. In addition, in our recent publication, we could show that the cholesterol transporter ABCA1 is deregulated in early-onset preeclampsia resulted from placental hypoxia [24, 25]. These results focused on the importance of the maternal-fetal cholesterol transport for adequate development of the fetus.

Microarray datasets of basal plate biopsies of both normal placentation and PE (24–36 weeks) demonstrated novel observations indicating increased expression of the leptin receptor Siglec-6 and pappalysin (PAPP-A2), a metalloproteinase that cleaves insulin-like growth factor (IGF)-binding protein-5 (IGFBP-5), in PE placentas compared to controls. Overall, these results suggest alterations in important biological processes including pathways that are regulated by leptin and IGF signals [9].

3. Early diagnosis

The aim for the early diagnosis is to start a preventive therapy by administration of 100 mg acetylsalicylic acid (ASS, aspirin) before 16 weeks of pregnancy (reduction of risk for severe preeclampsia: RR 0.1; 95% KI 0.1–0.74) [26]. It is clear that a risk calculation in the first trimester would be the most effective method to prevent preeclampsia.

Since the data on the usefulness of early administration of aspirin is still emerging, the optimal dose, which is probably 70–160 mg/d, is still under investigation. There is a known aspirin resistance in 33% of all women, which justifies the introduction of at least 100 instead of 80 mg aspirin/d. The combination of aspirin and low-molecular-weight heparin in secondary prevention seems to bring an additional benefit over aspirin alone [27], especially for an additional hereditary thrombophilia [28].

Early detection is based on three main points which are focused on and complement each other: a detailed medical history, the collection of biophysical parameters such as blood pressure, arterial stiffness, and Doppler examination of maternal blood vessels, and the determination of biochemical parameters, which can give clues to impaired placental function.

4. Maternal risk factors

The risk factors that are involved in the development of preeclampsia are also the symptoms of the metabolic syndrome and glucose metabolism disorders such as diabetes mellitus as well as insulin resistance and assisted reproductive techniques, increased body mass index (>35 kg/m^2), and increased diastolic blood pressure > 80 mm Hg [29]. Further risk factors are positive preeclampsia of genetic background, multiple pregnancy, pregnancy above the age of 40, previous kidney-related problem, and coagulation problems [30, 31].

Specifically, prevalent coagulation problems connected with high risk of preeclampsia is factor V Leiden mutation, homozygous MTHFR mutation, hyperhomocysteinemia, existence of antiphospholipid antibodies, and the mixture of multiple thrombophilias [32].

Immune system cause-related problems can be ascribed to the high risk, for instance, in the first pregnancy. In contrast, multiparity with the same partner has lower risk [33].

As to record, 30% of women with preeclampsia are identified early with inaccurate positive rate of 5% [29]. As to the pregnancy-generated hypertension without preeclampsia, the motherly record is much more important than the maternal serum parameters and pulsatility indices of uterine arteries [34].

5. Parameters in biophysics

Mean pressure of arterial blood in the first trimester can be implemented in pairs with risk factors of maternity as a predictor of preeclampsia in the first trimester that has a detection rate of 76% for early-onset preeclampsia. Systolic blood pressure is already substantially different in the first trimester regarding the early- and late-onset preeclampsia and pregnancy-generated hypertension [35].

The arterial supply to the uterus happens normally via uterine arteries, which change into circular running arteria arcuata. In this condition, the radial artery branches and spiral arteries move deeply into the myometrium and supply the decidua and fetus during pregnancy.

Anomalous placentation and incomplete cytotrophoblast invasion typified by inadequate formation and vasodilation of the spiral arteries have long been identified as one of the main risk factors for the growth of preeclampsia [36, 37].

These morphological changes indicate abnormal uteroplacental circulation typically characterized by a persistence of the postsystolic (Notch) and high resistance indices. A prediction of the severe form of pregnancy-induced hypertension and preeclampsia is possible by examining the uteroplacental vessels in the first and second trimesters. Various publications showed that in the first-trimester screening, Doppler examination of the uterine arteries identified a certain percentage of pregnant women that later develop preeclampsia with elevated uterine resistance indices and postsystolic incisions [38–40].

About 40% of pregnant women can thus be detected at a false-positive rate of 5% [34, 41]. However, the sensitivity for the prediction of preeclampsia is significantly lower than that in the second-trimester ultrasound measurements. Higher rates of sensitivity regarding the discovery of a late-onset preeclampsia can be achieved in the second trimester of pregnancy. Several Doppler studies in the second trimester yielded detection rates of 70–80% [42, 43].

6. Biochemical parameters

The problem of the Doppler examination alone, however, lies in the low predictive value. Only in combination with biochemical markers, this evaluation is clinically relevant for a preventive therapy. In the second trimester, the combination of Doppler sonography and angiogenic factors such as PlGF/sEndoglin (sEng) and sFlt-1 is a valid prediction of preeclampsia [44].

In order to intervene preventively, high-risk population should be identified before the 16th week of pregnancy. The aim is, therefore, to predict preeclampsia at the first trimester of pregnancy.

PAPP-A was first identified as a predictive marker. PlGF is also in the first quarter of pregnancy decreased. Further promising targets for the first-trimester screening are PP-13, soluble endoglin, inhibin A, activin A, pentraxin 3, P-selectin, IGFBP-1 and IGFBP-3, adiponectin, resistin, L-arginine, asymmetric dimethylarginine (ADMA), and homoarginine. However, sFlt-1 is not suitable for screening in the first trimester [34].

6.1 PIGF (placental growth factor)

PlGF belongs to the VEGF family, is secreted by trophoblast cells, and has proangiogenic function. Preeclampsia occurs due to an impaired placentation with subsequent ischemia triggers which raised secretion of antiangiogenic factors such as soluble Fms-like tyrosine kinase-1 (sFlt-1) and soluble endoglin (sEng) in the circulation of maternity. This process creates a course of antagonizing the angiogenic factors such as PlGF [45].

PIGF was in an early focus of the research groups in the search for a suitable prediction factor. It turned out that the concentration of PlGF in a preeclamptic pregnancy did not increase to the extent as would be expected in a normal pregnancy [46, 47]. Others could show that in the first trimester, there are already significant differences between PlGF concentrations in maternal blood of pregnant women with normal pregnancy and those that develop preeclampsia during pregnancy [34, 48–50]. Since 2011, the first conventional test of the company Alere allows the quantitative detection of PIGF in anticoagulated EDTA plasma in the first trimester with fluorescence immunoassay (sensitivity and specificity 95%). The detection rate of preeclampsia using PlGF alone for the early-onset preeclampsia is between 41 and 59% and for late-onset preeclampsia 33% [51].

The latest studies show a strong connection between changed levels of PlGF and sVEGF R1 in preeclamptic pregnancy, as well as in those who will eventually develop the condition later in pregnancy. These reports are based on the findings that sVEGF R1 levels increase earlier and to a greater extent in women who eventually develop preeclampsia compared to women with normal pregnancies. In contrast, free PlGF levels in women who develop preeclampsia (compared to women with normal pregnancies) are meaningfully lower. Latest data indicate these markers to be convincing in the differential examinations of hypertensive diseases of pregnancy [52, 53].

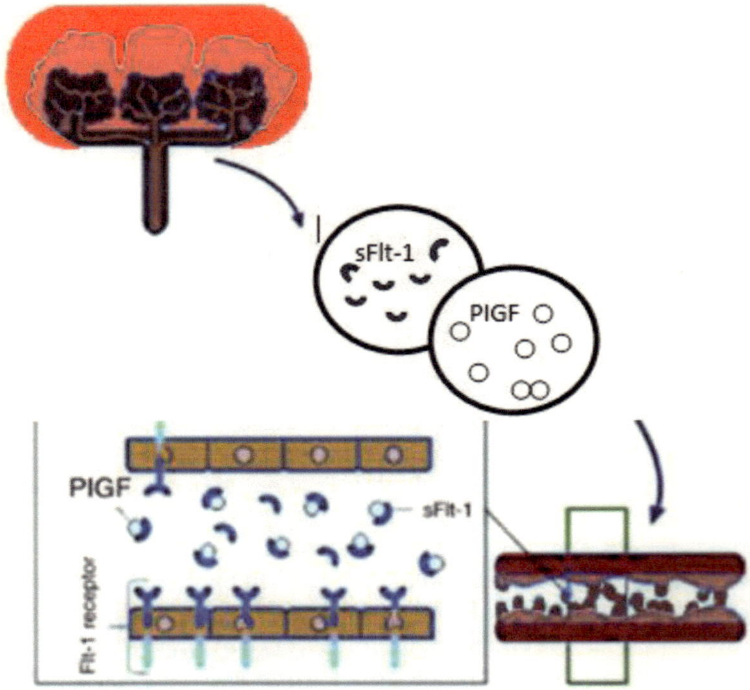

Figure 2.
An excessive production of sFlt-1 is known in patients with preeclampsia. As an antagonist, it binds with high affinity to free PIGF in maternal serum. Thereby, proangiogenic effects by binding of PIGF to membranous sFlt-1 receptors (a vascular endothelial growth factor) are inhibited and are thought to be responsible for endothelial dysfunction.

6.2 sFlt-1/PlGF ratio

Researches show that sFlt-1 is an antiangiogenic molecule and therefore seems to be involved importantly in the pathogenesis of preeclampsia. High levels of circulatings sFlt-1 in early pregnancy are associated with the later commencement of preeclampsia. An in vitro research shows that sFlt-1 inhibits tube formation of endothelial cells from human umbilical vein. In essential cytotrophoblast cell culture, sFlt-1 production and mRNA expression are related inversely to oxygen saturation. A twofold elevation in the level of sFlt-1 was also observed when normal villous explants were exposed to a hypoxic state (1% oxygen), compared with physiologic exposure to 5% oxygen. Therefore, it is reasonable that the hypoxic placenta releases an excess of sFlt-1 into the maternal circulation, which induces maternal endothelial dysfunction and clinical symptoms of preeclampsia. There is also a tendency that an excess of sFlt-1 production can trigger events in the pathogenesis of preeclampsia [55].

Especially, the sFlt-1/PlGF ratio connects to the clinical condition of the disease, differentiates between healthy and preeclamptic pregnancies, and gives a short-term prediction of disease development. Consequently, the estimation of sFlt-1 and PlGF was measured in clinical routine as a reliable and meaningful tool in examining and monitoring PE [56].

Research on antiangiogenesis factors such as sFlt-1 failed to convince as the exclusive marker for the prediction of preeclampsia in the first trimester [51]. Verlohren et al. showed that the combination of angiogenesis and antiangiogenesis factors, at least in the second and third trimesters, may offer the possibility of a risk classification by an sFlt-1/PlGF ratio. It was found that patients with preeclampsia had a significantly increased sFlt-1/PlGF ratio compared to patients with a normal pregnancy [16, 57, 58] (**Figure 2**).

6.3 PAPP-A

Pregnancy-associated plasma protein A (PAPP-A), an insulin-like growth factor-binding protein protease, is secreted by the syncytiotrophoblast. As part of the first-trimester screening, it has long been used in risk calculation for chromosomal abnormalities. We could show that patients with decreased levels of PAPP-A in maternal blood during the first trimester develop preeclampsia [54], especially an early-onset preeclampsia as revealed also by others [34, 59, 60, 74].

6.4 Inhibin A and activin A

Both glycoprotein hormones are produced by the fetoplacental unit. Several studies exhibited that both inhibin A and activin A are increased in the first trimester in maternal blood of patients who later develop preeclampsia compared to pregnant women with normal pregnancies [60, 61]. However, no association is found between impaired trophoblast invasion and subsequent endothelial dysfunction and increased concentration of activin A [62].

6.5 PP13

The placental protein 13 plays a role in physiological placentation. Because of impaired placentation in the presence of preeclampsia, there is an increased secretion of PP13 in the first trimester of pregnancy [63–67].

6.6 PTX3

Pentraxin 3 is a secreted protein as part of an inflammatory immune response and is increased as an acute phase protein molecule [62]. Both with manifestations of PE and before clinical symptoms, there is an increased secretion of PTX 3 in the maternal circulation [60, 68–70].

6.7 P-selectin

As a cell adhesion molecule, P-selectin plays a role in endothelial dysfunction. The consequence of placental ischemia in the context of preeclampsia is endothelial dysfunction and thus increased secretion of P-selectin [71]. This is already detectable in the first trimester of pregnancy [60, 69, 70].

6.8 IGFBP-1 and IGFBP-3

Both insulin-like growth factor-binding proteins are the focus of new research. Both in early- and late-onset preeclampsia, IGFBP-1 is decreased in the first trimester. Such changes are detected by secretion of IGFBP-3 only in late-onset preeclampsia. In both cases, there is no correlation to a disturbed trophoblast invasion [72, 73].

6.9 Adiponectin

In the case of early-onset PE, adiponectin levels are higher than in the first trimester compared to normal controls. This does not apply to late-onset PE. There is no relationship between adiponectin and PAPP-A levels and Doppler values. In addition, there is no advantage in prediction by the addition of adiponectin [75].

6.10 Resistin

Resistin levels in the first trimester are higher in patients who develop preeclampsia than controls. There is no relationship to impaired placental perfusion [75].

6.11 L-Arginine, asymmetric dimethylarginine (ADMA), and homoarginine

All three substances are part of NO metabolism. L-Arginine and L-homoarginine are increased in the first trimester at later-developing early-onset preeclampsia, as well as the ratio of ADMA/L-arginine and ADMA/L-homoarginine. This is not the case for late-onset preeclampsia and for the isolated analysis of ADMA [76].

7. Outlook

All biophysical and biochemical markers shown are used for prediction of preeclampsia. Meanwhile it has been obvious that a single diagnostic marker is not strong enough to accurately assume subsequent preeclampsia. Based on this reason, seemingly it is convincing to use historical, biophysical, and several biochemical parameters to ascertain the best possible detection rate is achieved.

Finally, one must distinguish between early- and late-onset preeclampsia in order to classify the present results correctly. The early-onset preeclampsia is defined as the onset before 34 weeks of pregnancy, the intermediate-onset preeclampsia between the 34 and 37 weeks, and the late-onset preeclampsia after 37 weeks. The late-onset PE seems to follow a different pathogenetic mechanism, since the serum parameters differ significantly as a marker of disturbed placentation in terms of predictive power [34]. The placentation disorder, according to previous published data, is a feature of early preeclampsia. The addition of biochemical markers in the first trimester is therefore particularly suitable for detection of early preeclampsia.

Poon et al. pioneered the evaluation of a few serum parameters and maternal factors in order to achieve a good predictive power of early preeclampsia. The detection rate of early-onset PE is 93.1% in the first trimester by algorithms from maternal risk factors, mean arterial blood pressure, pulsatility index of the uterine arteries, PAPP-A, and PlGF. The detection rate for the late-onset PE with an appropriate algorithm is 44.9% [34].

These named parameters can now be purchased commercially and combined with appropriate software. Akolekar et al. found that the detection rate of preeclampsia in the first trimester by a combination of several markers (PIGF, PAPP-A, PP13, inhibin A, activin A, sEndoglin, PTX3, P-selectin, blood pressure, Doppler sonography, and history) is increased significantly to a detection rate of 91% at a fixed 5% false-positive rate for early-onset PE, 79.4% for intermediate-onset PE (34–37th weeks of gestation), and 60% for late-onset PE [60]. The addition of these parameters allows a better predictive power of all forms of preeclampsia compared to the above-described relatively simple algorithm, having particular effect on a high detection rate for early-onset preeclampsia.

Further studies are expected that show which of the biochemical markers are really useful in clinical practice. The relation of costs and benefit must be explored.

Finally, the question arises that how far it may succeed in establishing the first-trimester screening tests with the consecutive possible prevention by aspirin and/or low-molecular-weight heparin, as a screening in a large, unselected collective. Since prevention is simple and inexpensive, the obstacle is much more on a personal and cost-intensive screening tool. The investigation regarding chromosome abnormalities will depend on the basis of the consequences of abnormal test results of many factors and is always carried out only in a preselected group. Examining on preeclampsia should be for a much larger group of pregnant women, not at least because of the higher risk to get preeclampsia as a chromosomal abnormal baby and the simplicity of prophylaxis. The other essential reason for early preeclampsia risk estimation is the fact that preeclamptic pregnant women have a bigger lifetime risk for suffering heart and blood vessel disease. Better observation of this collective of patients, changing of lifestyle factors, and health education could be an important step to reduce morbidity and mortality according to cardiovascular problems worldwide.

Currently, the aspect of fetal programming is in the main focus of research. Not only the mother also the offspring bears the consequences of preeclamptic pregnancy with mostly intrauterine growth restriction like elevated risk for cardiovascular diseases and behavioral disorders, for example.

It would be desirable in the future to integrate preeclampsia risk calculation to the regular prenatal care in the first trimester. Further studies on large collectives have to determine to what extent the false-positive and false-negative findings can lead in relation to health and economic disadvantages. Even an early screening should not replace careful pregnancy monitoring.

Finally, pregnancy is not only a short time in a woman's life with the aim to deliver a baby but it is also an important time giving insights in women's health status. As we already know, pregnancy may positively influence women's health future as could be shown by studies which detected a reduced risk of developing breast cancer after pregnancy. As an indicator of risk factors, pregnancy is not only the beginning of taking care for a family but also for a better self-care [77].

8. Conclusion

To conclude, the best possible detection rate of preeclampsia seems to be convincing to apply historical, biophysical, and several biochemical parameters. A detailed medical history such as diabetes mellitus, assisted reproductive techniques, increase body mass index, family background, multiple pregnancy, pregnancy over 40 years, previous renal problem, and clotting disorder. The collection of biophysical parameters such as blood pressure, arterial stiffness, and Doppler examination of maternal blood vessels. The determination of biochemical parameter such as angiogenic factors PIGF, sFlt-1, PAPP-A, inhibin A, activin A, PP13, PTX3, P-selectin, IGFBP-1 and IGFBP-3, adiponectin, resistin, L-arginine, ADMA, and homoarginine.

Author details

Makmur Sitepu* and Jusuf Rachmadsyah
Department of Obstetric and Gynecology, Medical Faculty, Universitas Sumatera Utara, Medan, Indonesia

*Address all correspondence to: makmurstp@gmail.com

References

[1] Villar K. Eclampsia and pre-eclampsia: A health problem for 2000 years. In: Critchley H, MacLean A, Poston L, editors. Preeclampsia. London, UK: RCOG Press; 2003. pp. 189-207

[2] Noris M, Perico N, Remuzzi G. Mechanisms of disease: Pre-eclampsia. Nature Clinical Practice Nephrology. 2005;**1**(2):98-120

[3] Barker DJP, Osmond C, Forsen TJ, Kajantie E, Eriksson JG. Maternal and social origins of hypertension. Hypertension. 2007;**50**(3):565-571

[4] Barker DJP. Intrauterine programming of adult disease. Molecular Medicine Today. 1995;**1**(9):418-423

[5] Godfrey KM, Inskip HM, Hanson MA. The long-term effects of prenatal development on growth and metabolism. Seminars in Reproductive Medicine. 2011;**29**(3):257-265. (PMC free article)

[6] Cross JC, Baczyk D, Dobric N, et al. Genes, development and evolution of the placenta. Placenta. 2003;**24**(2-3):123-130

[7] Roberts JM, Cooper DW. Pathogenesis and genetics of pre-eclampsia. The Lancet. 2001;**357**(9249):53-56

[8] Redman CW, Sargent IL. Latest advances in understanding preeclampsia. Science. 2005;**308**(5728):1592-1594

[9] Winn VD, Gormley M, Fisher SJ. The impact of preeclampsia on gene expression at the maternal-fetal interface. Pregnancy Hypertension. 2011;**1**(1):100-108. (PMC free article)

[10] Zhou Y, Damsky CH, Chiu K, Roberts JM, Fisher SJ. Preeclampsia is associated with abnormal expression of adhesion molecules by invasive cytotrophoblasts. Journal of Clinical Investigation. 1993;**91**(3):950-960

[11] Kusanovic JP, Romero R, Chaiworapongsa T, et al. A prospective cohort study of the value of maternal plasma concentrations of angiogenic and anti-angiogenic factors in early pregnancy and midtrimester in the identification of patients destined to develop preeclampsia. Journal of Maternal-Fetal and Neonatal Medicine. 2009;**22**(11):1021-1038

[12] Stillman IE, Karumanchi SA. The glomerular injury of preeclampsia. Journal of the American Society of Nephrology. 2007;**18**(8):2281-2284

[13] Rolfo A, Many A, Racano A, et al. Abnormalities in oxygen sensing define early and late onset preeclampsia as distinct pathologies. PLoS One. 2010;**5**(10):e13288

[14] Banks RE, Forbes MA, Searles J, et al. Evidence for the existence of a novel pregnancy-associated soluble variant of the vascular endothelial growth factor receptor, Flt-1. Molecular Human Reproduction. 1998;**4**(4):377-386

[15] Verheul HMW, Pinedo HM. Possible molecular mechanisms involved in the toxicity of angiogenesis inhibition. Nature Reviews Cancer. 2007;**7**(6):475-485

[16] Verlohren S, Herraiz I, Lapaire O, et al. The sFlt-1/PlGF ratio in different types of hypertensive pregnancy disorders and its prognostic potential in preeclamptic patients. American Journal of Obstetrics & Gynecology. 2012;**206**(1):58.e1-58.e8

[17] Rana S, Powe CE, Salahuddin S, et al. Angiogenic factors and the risk of adverse outcomes in women with suspected preeclampsia. Circulation. 2012;**125**(7):911-919. (PMC free article)

[18] Perni U, Sison C, Sharma V, et al. Angiogenic factors in superimposed preeclampsia: A longitudinal study of women with chronic hypertension

during pregnancy. Hypertension. 2012;**59**(3):740-746

[19] Rajakumar A, Cerdeira AS, Rana S, et al. Transcriptionally active syncytial aggregates in the maternal circulation may contribute to circulating soluble fms-like tyrosine kinase 1 in preeclampsia. Hypertension. 2012;**59**(2):256-264. (PMC free article)

[20] Gellhaus A, Schmidt M, Dunk C, Lye SJ, Kimmig R, Winterhager E. Decreased expression of the angiogenic regulators CYR61 (CCN1) and NOV (CCN3) in human placenta is associated with pre-eclampsia. Molecular Human Reproduction. 2006;**12**(6):389-399

[21] Gellhaus A, Schmidt M, Dunk C, Lye SJ, Winterhager E. The circulating proangiogenic factors CYR61 (CCN1) and NOV (CCN3) are significantly decreased in placentae and sera of preeclamptic patients. Reproductive Sciences. 2007;**14**(8):46-52

[22] Wolf N, Yang W, Dunk CE, et al. Regulation of the matricellular proteins CYR61 (CCN1) and NOV (CCN3) by hypoxia-inducible factor-1α and transforming-growth factor-β3 in the human trophoblast. Endocrinology. 2010;**151**(6):2835-2845

[23] Yang W, Wagener J, Gellhaus A. Impact of CCN3 (NOV) glycosylation on migration/invasion properties and cell growth of the choriocarcinoma cell line Jeg3. Human Reproduction. 2011;**26**(10):2850-2860

[24] Plösch T, Gellhaus A, van Straten EM, et al. The liver X receptor, (LXR) and its target gene ABCA1 are regulated upon low oxygen in human trophoblast cells: A reason for alterations in preeclampsia? Placenta. 2010;**31**(10):910-918

[25] Ugocsai P, Hohenstatt A, Paragh G, et al. HIF-1β determines ABCA1 expression under hypoxia in human macrophages. International Journal of Biochemistry and Cell Biology. 2010;**42**(2):241-252

[26] Bujold E, Morency AM, Roberge S, Lacasse Y, Forest JC, Giguère Y. Acetylsalicylic acid for the prevention of preeclampsia and intra-uterine growth restriction in women with abnormal uterine artery Doppler: A systematic review and meta-analysis. Journal of Obstetrics and Gynaecology Canada. 2009;**31**(9):818-826

[27] Gris JC, Chauleur C, Molinari N, et al. Addition of enoxaparin to aspirin for the secondary prevention of placental vascular complications in women with severe pre-eclampsia. The pilot randomized controlled NOH-PE trial. Thrombosis and Haemostasis. 2011;**106**(6):1053-1061

[28] deVries JI, van Pampus MG, Hague WM, Bezemer PD, Joosten JH. FRUIT investigators. Low-molecular-weight heparin added to aspirin in the prevention of recurrent early-onset preeclampsia in women with inheritable thrombophilia: The FRUIT-RCT. Journal of Thrombosis and Haemostasis. 2012;**10**(1):64-72

[29] Yu CKH, Smith GCS, Papageorghiou AT, Cacho AM, Nicolaides KH. An integrated model for the prediction of preeclampsia using maternal factors and uterine artery Doppler velocimetry in unselected low-risk women. American Journal of Obstetrics and Gynecology. 2005;**193**(2):429-436

[30] Sibai B, Dekker G, Kupferminc M. Pre-eclampsia. The Lancet. 2005;**365**(9461):785-799

[31] Steegers EAP, von Dadelszen P, Duvekot JJ, Pijnenborg R. Pre-eclampsia. The Lancet. 2010;**376**(9741):631-644

[32] Benedetto C, Marozio L, Tavella AM, Salton L, Grivon S, Di Giampaolo F. Coagulation disorders in pregnancy: Acquired and inherited thrombophilias.

Annals of the New York Academy of Sciences. 2010;**1205**:106-117

[33] Skjaerven R, Wilcox AJ, Lie RT. The interval between pregnancies and the risk of preeclampsia. The New England Journal of Medicine. 2002;**346**(1):33-38

[34] Poon LCY, Staboulidou I, Maiz N, Plasencia W, Nicolaides KH. Hypertensive disorders in pregnancy: Screening by uterine artery Doppler at 11-13 weeks. Ultrasound in Obstetrics and Gynecology. 2009;**34**(2):142-148

[35] Poon LCY, Kametas NA, Valencia C, Chelemen T, Nicolaides KH. Hypertensive disorders in pregnancy: Screening by systolic diastolic and mean arterial pressure at 11-13 weeks. Hypertension in Pregnancy. 2011;**30**(1):93-107

[36] Brosens IA, Robertson WB, Dixon HG. The role of spiral arteries in the pathogenesis of preeclampsia. In: Wynn RM, editor. Obstetrics and Gynecology Annual. New York, NY, USA: Appleton-Century-Crafts; 1972. pp. 177-191

[37] Pijnenborg R, Vercruysse L, Hanssens M. The uterine spiral arteries in human pregnancy: Facts and controversies. Placenta. 2006;**27**(9-10):939-958

[38] Lovgren TR, Dugoff L, Galan HL. Uterine artery Doppler and prediction of preeclampsia. Clinical Obstetrics and Gynecology. 2010;**53**(4):888-898

[39] Bahado-Singh RO, Jodicke C. Uterine artery Doppler in first-trimester pregnancy screening. Clinical Obstetrics and Gynecology. 2010;**53**(4):879-887

[40] Carbillon L. First trimester uterine artery Doppler for the prediction of preeclampsia and foetal growth restriction. Journal of Maternal-Fetal and Neonatal Medicine. 2012;**25**(7):877-883

[41] Cuckle HS. Screening for pre-eclampsia-lessons from aneuploidy screening. Placenta. 2011;**32**(supplement 1):S42-S48

[42] Costa F, Murthi P, Keogh R, Woodrow N. Early screening for preeclampsia. Revista Brasileira de Ginecologia e Obstetrícia. 2011;**33**(11):367-375

[43] Pedrosa AC, Matias A. Screening for pre-eclampsia: A systematic review of tests combining uterine artery Doppler with other markers. Journal of Perinatal Medicine. 2011;**39**(6):619-635

[44] Stepan H, Geipel A, Schwarz F, Krämer T, Wessel N, Faber R. Circulatory soluble endoglin and its predictive value for preeclampsia in second-trimester pregnancies with abnormal uterine perfusion. American Journal of Obstetrics and Gynecology. 2008;**198**(2):175.e1-175.e6

[45] Lockwood CJ, Krikun G, Caze R, Rahman M, Buchwalder LF, Schatz F. Decidual cell-expressed tissue factor in human pregnancy and its involvement in hemostasis and preeclampsia-related angiogenesis. Annals of the New York Academy of Sciences. 2008;**1127**:67-72

[46] Schmidt M, Dogan C, Birdir C, et al. Altered angiogenesis in preeclampsia: Evaluation of a new test system for measuring placental growth factor. Clinical Chemistry and Laboratory Medicine. 2007;**45**(11):1504-1510

[47] Schmidt M, Dogan C, Birdir C, et al. Placental growth factor: A predictive marker for preeclampsia? Gynakologisch-geburtshilflicheRundschau. 2009;**49**(2):94-99

[48] Akolekar R, Zaragoza E, Poon LCY, Pepes S, Nicolaides KH. Maternal serum placental growth factor at 11 + 0 to 13 + 6 weeks of gestation in the prediction of pre-eclampsia. Ultrasound in Obstetrics and Gynecology. 2008;**32**(6):732-739

[49] Vatten LJ, Eskild A, Nilsen TIL, Jeansson S, Jenum PA, Staff AC. Changes in circulating level of angiogenic factors from the first to second trimester as predictors of preeclampsia. American Journal of Obstetrics and Gynecology. 2007;**196**(3):239.e1-239.e6

[50] Rana S, Karumanchi SA, Levine RJ, et al. Sequential changes in antiangiogenic factors in early pregnancy and risk of developing preeclampsia. Hypertension. 2007;**50**(1):137-142

[51] Kuc S, Wortelboer EJ, van Rijn BB, Franx A, Visser GHA, Schielen PCJI. Evaluation of 7 serum biomarkers and uterine artery Doppler ultrasound for first-trimester prediction of preeclampsia: A systematic review. Obstetrical and Gynecological Survey. 2011;**66**(4):225-239

[52] Sunderji S, Gaziano E, Wothe D, Rogers LC, Sibai B, Karumanchi SA, et al. Automated assays for sVEGF R1 and PlGF as an aid in the diagnosis of preterm preeclampsia: A prospective clinical study. American Journal of Obstetrics and Gynecology. 2010;**202**(1):40-e1

[53] Chaiworapongsa T, Romero R, Kim YM, Kim GJ, Kim MR, Espinoza J, et al. Plasma soluble vascular endothelial growth factor receptor-1 concentration is elevated prior to the clinical diagnosis of pre-eclampsia. The Journal of Maternal-Fetal & Neonatal Medicine. 2005;**17**(1):3-18

[54] Mikat B, Zeller A, Scherag A, et al. βhCG and PAPP-A in first trimester: Predictive factors for preeclampsia? Hypertension in Pregnancy. 2012;**31**(2):261-267

[55] Lu F, Longo M, Tamayo E, Maner W, Al-Hendy A, Anderson GD, et al. The effect of over-expression of sFlt-1 on blood pressure and the occurrence of other manifestations of preeclampsia in unrestrained conscious pregnant mice. American Journal of Obstetrics and Gynecology. 2007;**196**(4):396.e1-396.e7

[56] Spencer K, Cowans NJ, Nicolaides KH. Low levels of maternal serum PAPP-A in the first trimester and the risk of pre-eclampsia. Prenatal Diagnosis. 2008;**28**(1):7-10

[57] Shibata E, Rajakumar A, Powers RW, Larkin RW, Gilmour C, Bodnar LM, et al. Soluble fms-like tyrosine kinase 1 is increased in preeclampsia but not in normotensive pregnancies with small-for-gestational-age neonates: Relationship to circulating placental growth factor. The Journal of Clinical Endocrinology & Metabolism. 2005;**90**(8):4895-4903

[58] Ohkuchi A, Hirashima C, Suzuki H, Takahashi K, Yoshida M, Matsubara S, et al. Evaluation of a new and automated electrochemiluminescence immunoassay for plasma sFlt-1 and PlGF levels in women with preeclampsia. Hypertension Research. 2010;**33**(5):422

[59] Ossada V, Jank A, Stepan H. The impact of uterine curettage postpartum on maternal sFlt-1 concentration. Journal of Perinatal Medicine. 2016;**44**(3):351-354

[60] Akolekar R, Syngelaki A, Sarquis R, Zvanca M, Nicolaides KH. Prediction of early, intermediate and late pre-eclampsia from maternal factors, biophysical and biochemical markers at 11-13 weeks. Prenatal Diagnosis. 2011;**31**(1):66-74

[61] Akolekar R, Etchegaray A, Zhou Y, Maiz N, Nicolaides KH. Maternal serum activin A at 11-13 weeks of gestation in hypertensive disorders of pregnancy. Fetal Diagnosis and Therapy. 2009;**25**(3):320-327

[62] Akolekar R, Minekawa R, Veduta A, Romero XC, Nicolaides KH. Maternal plasma inhibin A at 11-13 weeks of gestation in hypertensive disorders of pregnancy. Prenatal Diagnosis. 2009;**29**(8):753-760

[63] Huppertz B, Sammar M, Chefetz I, Neumaier-Wagner P, Bartz C, Meiri H. Longitudinal determination of serum placental protein 13 during development of preeclampsia. Fetal Diagnosis and Therapy. 2008;**24**(3):230-236

[64] Khalil A, Cowans NJ, Spencer K, Goichman S, Meiri H, Harrington K. First trimester maternal serum placental protein 13 for the prediction of pre-eclampsia in women with a priori high risk. Prenatal Diagnosis. 2009;**29**(8):781-789

[65] Chafetz I, Kuhnreich I, Sammar M, et al. First-trimester placental protein 13 screening for preeclampsia and intrauterine growth restriction. American Journal of Obstetrics and Gynecology. 2007;**197**(1):35.e1-37.e1

[66] Spencer K, Cowans NJ, Chefetz I, Tal J, Meiri H. First-trimester maternal serum PP-13, PAPP-A and second-trimester uterine artery Doppler pulsatility index as markers of pre-eclampsia. Ultrasound in Obstetrics and Gynecology. 2007;**29**(2):128-134

[67] Burger O, Pick E, Zwickel J, et al. Placental protein 13 (PP-13): Effects on cultured trophoblasts, and its detection in human body fluids in normal and pathological pregnancies. Placenta. 2004;**25**(7):608-622

[68] Garlanda C, Bottazzi B, Bastone A, Mantovani A. Pentraxins at the crossroads between innate immunity, inflammation, matrix deposition, and female fertility. Annual Review of Immunology. 2005;**23**:337-366

[69] Poon LCY, Akolekar R, Lachmann R, Beta J, Nicolaides KH. Hypertensive disorders in pregnancy: Screening by biophysical and biochemical markers at 11-13 weeks. Ultrasound in Obstetrics and Gynecology. 2010;**35**(6):662-670

[70] Poon LCY, Stratieva V, Piras S, Piri S, Nicolaides KH. Hypertensive disorders in pregnancy: Combined screening by uterine artery Doppler, blood pressure and serum PAPP-A at 11-13 weeks. Prenatal Diagnosis. 2010;**30**(3):216-223

[71] Granger JP, Alexander BT, Llinas MT, Bennett WA, Khalil RA. Pathophysiology of hypertension during preeclampsia linking placental ischemia with endothelial dysfunction. Hypertension. 2001;**38**(3):718-722

[72] Sifakis S, Akolekar R, Kappou D, Mantas N, Nicolaides KH. Maternal serum insulin-like growth factor-binding protein-1 (IGFBP-1) at 11-13 weeks in pre-eclampsia. Prenatal Diagnosis. 2011;**31**(2):196-201

[73] Sifakis S, Akolekar R, Kappou D, Mantas N, Nicolaides KH. Maternal serum insulin-like growth factor-binding protein-3 (IGFBP-3) at 11-13 weeks in pre-eclampsia. Journal of Human Hypertension. 2012;**26**(4):253-258

[74] Nanda S, Yu CKH, Giurcaneanu L, Akolekar R, Nicolaides KH. Maternal serum adiponectin at 11-13 weeks of gestation in preeclampsia. Fetal Diagnosis and Therapy. 2011;**29**(3):208-215

[75] Nanda S, Poon LCY, Muhaisen M, Acosta IC, Nicolaides KH. Maternal serum resistin at 11 to 13 weeks' gestation in normal and pathological pregnancies. Metabolism. 2012;**61**(5):699-705

[76] Khalil AA, Tsikas D, Akolekar R, Jordan J, Nicolaides KH. Asymmetric dimethylarginine, arfinine and homoarginine at 11-13 weeks gestation andpreeclampsia: A case-control study. Journal of Human Hypertension. Jan 2013;**27**(1):38-43. In press

[77] Ives A, Saunders C, Bulsara M, Semmens J. Pregnancy after breast cancer: Population based study. British Medical Journal. 2007;**334**(7586):194-196

Section 2

The Etiology and Prediction in Segregated Populations

Chapter 3

Placental Adaptation to Hypoxia as a Predictive Marker for Preeclampsia

Sarah I.Y. Ahmed

Abstract

The ability of the placenta to interact with surrounding microenvironment of hypoxia can serve as a predictive marker for the development of preeclampsia. Lessons can be studied from highlands inhabitants and their ability to survive extreme conditions of hypobaric hypoxia. Many candidate genes loci that are associated with adaptation to high altitude hypoxia and healthy exercise are also associated with adaptation to hypoxia in normal pregnancy. This can pave the way to a new approach based on the concept of evolution and adaptation stating that "genes can undergo a process of natural selection for the fittest adaptive variants, so as to reach a state of adaptation to the scarce microenvironments." Accordingly, the degree of adaptation in candidate genes and their polymorphisms can serve as predictive markers for the development of preeclampsia. This can be seen in the high degree of concordance between gene expression and the lesions seen in the placenta and other remote organs in the different subtypes of preeclampsia. To conclude, "adaptive or less adaptive" can be the genetic result that answers the question of disease prediction, recurrence, and possible complications.

Keywords: placenta, adaptation, hypoxia, predictive marker

1. Introduction

Throughout the lives of individuals, their genes interact with their environments to cause variations in phenotype traits. Because individuals with certain traits tend to survive and reproduce more than others with less successful traits, the population evolves. In 1859, Charles Darwin set out his theory of evolution by natural selection as an explanation for adaptation and speciation. He defined natural selection as the "principle by which each slight variation [of a trait], if useful, is preserved" [1]. Although the Darwinian theory was ages before the genome era, it can also explain the process of natural selection at molecular levels; cells with successful traits are best adapted to their microenvironments, and more likely to survive and proliferate. The selection between cells favors those with the most advantageous genetic polymorphisms. The genetic variability is usually enhanced by the scarce microenvironments like low oxygen, low temperature, and high radiation that act as competitive milieus for cells. The useful genetic variants are preserved and can be heritable.

Some 2.4 billion years ago, photosynthesis leads to the accumulation of oxygen to levels that were likely toxic to many microorganisms. Organisms that could

IntechOpen

defend themselves against oxidative stress and at the same time utilize oxygen for energy, survived and evolved. As time went on, cellular requirement for oxygen became critical, and animals developed a physiological response to the low levels of oxygen. The cellular ability to compete in such scarce microenvironments became the "microevolutionary" exam for survival in many physiological processes as in hematopoiesis, spermatogenesis, normal pregnancy, and embryogenesis. Genetic studies suggest that hypoxia-inducible factors (HIFs) are a family of master transcriptional regulators for the hypoxic response inside the body. HIF-α transcription factors (HIF-1α and HIF-2α/EPAS1) dimerize with HIF-1β/ARNT subunits, and translocate to the nucleus, where it binds to the hypoxia responsive element (HRE) in the genetic material to regulate the transcription of some 200 genes, leading to the adaptive response to hypoxic stress. In turn, hypoxia responsive genes promote the tolerance of hypoxia by decreasing the cellular requirement for oxygen and increasing the supply of oxygen. They mainly involved in angiogenesis, erythropoiesis, energy metabolism, and autophagy [2].

On ascent to high attitudes, lowlanders become at risk of conditions like acute mountain sickness (AMS), pulmonary edema, cerebral edema, and polycythemia in the chronic type of the disease. These conditions, which resemble many symptoms associated with preeclampsia, are considered to be a maladaptive response to the low oxygen levels at high altitudes. However, ancient indigenous populations like Tibetans through generations acquired unique integrated physiological processes for defending their body against oxygen deprivation. This gives them the advantage of being protected from hypoxia-related disorders, like hypertension, diabetes mellitus, cardiovascular disorders, and preeclampsia. Yet, physiological acclimatization can occur in lowlanders over days to weeks following ascent and can serve as the first steps of adaptation. This led to the idea that adaptation to hypoxia can also protect from pathological disorders that result in dysregulation of hypoxia pathways like in preeclampsia [3].

2. Preeclampsia as a maladaptive disorder

In spite of the extensive research in the pathophysiology of the disease, the etiology is still poorly understood. It was suggested to be due to the insufficient adaptation of spiral arterioles or due to the shallow trophoblastic invasion, resulting in reduced uteroplacental blood flow leading to placental hypoxia. The placenta initially develops in a low oxygen environment of 1–2% oxygen until after the 10th week of pregnancy. This maternal hypoxia is an effective stimulus eliciting adaptations at the maternal-fetal interface, which include activation of the invasive endovascular trophoblast cell lineage and modifications of uterine blood vessels supplying the developing chorioallantoic placenta. Reduced or absent cytotrophoblast invasion of the maternal uterine spiral arterioles is a common clinical finding in studies of pregnancies complicated by preeclampsia, suggesting that the mechanism mediating invasion of these cells is perturbed. While, it is proposed that hypoxia-inducible factors are the key regulators of the first trimester [4–7].

The exposure of pregnant women to hypobaric hypoxia at high altitudes leads to arterial maternal hypoxia and intervillous blood hypoxia at the maternal-fetal interface. This renders pregnant women from low-altitude to be at risk of many complications including reproductive loss, intrauterine growth restriction, and preeclampsia. However, high-altitude residents have low rates of preeclampsia compared to other populations at the same altitudes. Such population differences are due, at least in part, to differences in maternal vascular responses to pregnancy. It was hypothesized that natural selection acting on hypoxia-inducible factor

(HIF)-targeted or -regulatory genes has enabled maternal vascular adaptation to pregnancy in long-resident high-altitude groups. Earlier studies support this hypothesis and demonstrate that the potent genes can be differentially regulated between adaptive and less adaptive populations. Moore et al. show that HIF-targeted vasoconstrictor, endothelin-1 (ET-1), is differentially regulated by pregnancy in Andean vs. European residents at high altitudes. Andeans, who live longer at high altitude, show normal, pregnancy-associated fall in ET-1 levels; whereas, Europeans have higher ET-1 levels and little pregnancy-associated change, like in preeclamptic women. Another hopeful study revealed that high-altitude Tibetans, who have lived the longest at high altitude, can share similar genotypic and allelic frequencies of adaptive variants with sea level Sojourners who undergo acclimatization on ascent [8–10].

This led to the question that, if lowlanders on ascent have the ability to acquire allele and genotype frequency as in adaptive native individuals, can preeclamptic women undergo acclimatization, and can it be used as a predictive marker for the disease.

3. From preeclampsia to normal pregnancy: the hidden adaptation!

There are a very large number of both prospective and retrospective studies investigating the preeclampsia recurrence rate, with different sample sizes, target populations, study designs, and main outcome measures, resulting in contrasting conclusions. Yet, maternal and perinatal outcomes in the subsequent pregnancy are generally better than in the first; most women will not have recurrent preeclampsia, and those who do usually will give birth at a greater gestational age compared with their index birth. Even though, women who have experienced a pregnancy complicated by preeclampsia, including their caregivers, undoubtedly have a fear of recurrence and should be counseled about their reproductive future. Many of these mothers and babies are at increased risk of severe adverse outcomes that include acute renal or hepatic failure, antepartum and postpartum hemorrhage, stroke, maternal death, intrauterine growth restriction, and perinatal death. Long-term, the burden of preterm birth is immense, particularly in terms of neurodevelopmental impairment, impaired learning, cerebral palsy, and need for special care resources [11].

Another evidence for the hidden adaptation is the ability of the placenta to survive the oxidative stress. Uterine artery Doppler studies are proposed to be abnormal in the second trimester of pregnancy because of increased vascular resistance indicating failed remodeling of the vessels of the intervillous space. About half of women with abnormal uterine artery Doppler findings go on to have preeclampsia, preterm birth, or pregnancies complicated by IUGR, while, the other half go on to normal outcomes. Besides to the Doppler scans, biochemical markers, like reduced circulating ascorbate, increased concentrations of nitric oxide synthase, and AT1 angiotensin receptor inhibitors, show evidence of oxidative stress both in women with or without abnormal uterine artery velocimetry. These markers are present regardless of whether the pregnancy proceeds to IUGR, preeclampsia, or a normal outcome.

These findings support the concept that poor placentation (Stage 1 of the model) alone is not sufficient to cause preeclampsia, and that there are other factors that adjust the physiological wheel of oxidative stress toward adaptation and normal pregnancy or toward preeclampsia (stage 2 of the model) [12]. In other words, it appears that the placenta starts as preeclamptic, and then somehow overcomes the oxidative stress and continues the placentation normally. This raises many questions on what are the hidden mechanisms that enable the placenta to survive the oxidative stress and overcome the disease? What could happen in a subsequent pregnancy that renders them to be protected? Why the placenta from normal pregnancies survives the oxidative stress?

4. Hypoxia and natural selection

It is known that hypoxic microenvironment acts as a stress-induced mutagenesis by increasing genetic instability in human cell through highly regulated genetic mechanisms. The stabilization of HIF, the master transcriptional factor in hypoxia, down-regulates the major DNA repair mechanisms; mismatch repair and homologous recombination. This leads to a switch from the high-fidelity repair mechanisms to the error-prone mutagenic non-homologous end joining mechanisms, which result in a high degree of genetic variability. In earlier study, our findings revealed that genetic variability in periods of high hypoxic pressure in preeclamptic samples was more confined to certain genomic loci, in particular the HIF master regulators of hypoxia, compared to normal pregnancy [3, 13].

Different scenarios of genetic variability under stressful condition of hypoxia are proposed, and represent the basis for natural selection and adaptation. **Figure 1** shows

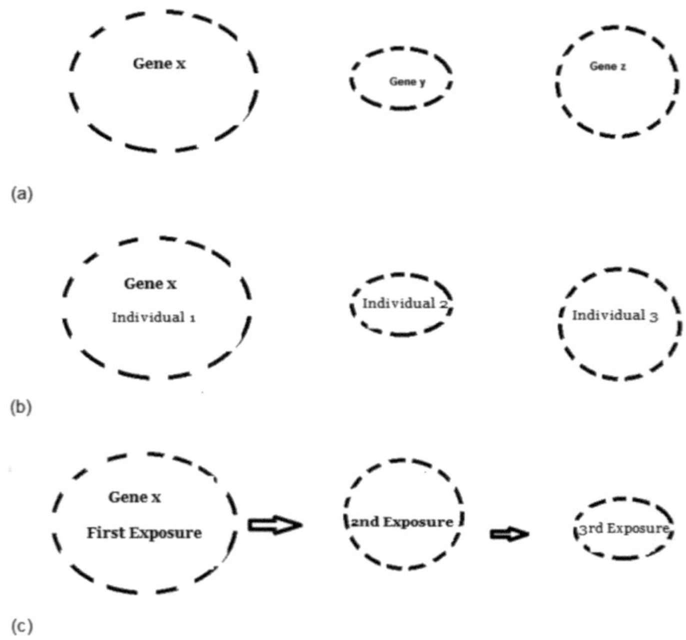

Figure 1.
The degree to which the genes can be reprogrammed by mutations can be termed genetic flexibility [14]. Genetic variability permits flexibility and survival of a population in the changing environments. Here, the genetic variability is represented by circles. The dots in the circles are the number of genetic variants in a particular gene. The more the variants are, the highest is the genetic flexibility. (a) Different genes in the same individual with the same degree of stressful condition. Gene x shows a larger circle with more variants, and this may indicates that gene x is more influential at a particular stressful condition, and probably is more affected by the signals of that particular condition. (b) The same gene in different individuals under the same extreme condition. Individual 1 with a larger circle of genetic variability is more flexible and have higher chance to adapt under the certain condition than 2 and 3. Individuals 2 and 3 are either less flexible due to different reasons, or (c) may undergo a previous acclimatization experience that renders them to show a less degree of variability. In (c), gene x is in the same individual, but the larger circle is showing genetic variants in the first exposure to stressful microenvironment (hypoxia), followed by the second, and the third exposure. The decrease in the number of genetic variants in subsequent exposures reflects the stress relief, and probably acclimatization.

dotted circles that represent the flexibility of hypoxia pathway genes under stressful conditions. The dots represent the genetic variants or mutations. The more flexible the gene is, the larger the circle of genetic variability, and thus the higher chances for natural selection to the fittest variants. This can predict the possible path of evolutionary events, and the possible roles of the genes with larger circles under stressful conditions.

In a previous report, we showed that preeclamptic samples had higher genetic variability in the key regulators of hypoxia pathway genes like EPAS1 and EGLN1 compared to normal pregnancy, which indicates that they were under a high level of stress. We also hypothesized that the high genetic variability that are reflected by the high number of mutations in preeclamptic samples can be considered as a "positive response" toward adaptation by increasing the chance of having adaptive mutations, yet they are still evolutionary late compared to controls. In other words, normal pregnancy has higher rate of fixation to the adaptive variants compared to preeclampsia, and this can be the reason for the delay in the process of adaptation in some types of preeclampsia [3].

5. Genetic association studies and preeclampsia

Genome-wide linkage studies of preeclampsia and pregnancy-induced hypertension have identified different loci associated with preeclampsia that segregate with different populations: on 4q (between D4S450-D4S610 markers, found in Australia), 2q23 (between D2S112-D2S151 markers, Australia, NZ), 2p13 (D2S286, Iceland), 2p25 (D2S168, Finland), 9p13 (D9S169, Finland), and 10q22 (Netherlands). Additional loci are expected to exist in preeclamptic patients with certain complications, such as the locus 12q in patients with hemolysis, elevated liver enzymes, and low platelets (HELLP) syndrome [15–18].

Candidate genes studies have provided evidence for an association with preeclampsia, frequently with inconsistent results. One of the common candidate genes is endothelial nitric oxide synthase gene (eNOS) on 7q36, which is responsible for nitric oxide production in endothelial cells. The endothelial dysfunction in preeclampsia reveals a strong association with eNOS polymorphisms. However, several other genome scans could not confirm this association. Another study found an evidence of moderate association with an increased risk for preeclampsia in women having mutations in coagulation factor genes; F5 Leiden (rs6025, G1691A), and the prothrombin (F2) gene (rs1799963, G20210A). This evidence may explain the association of the disease with coagulation disorders. Several studies found associations between renin-angiotensin-aldosterone system with gestational hypertension and preeclampsia. Earlier linkage studies found an association with angiotensinogen (AGT) locus, on 1q42-43 and the risk for hypertensive disease in different sets of population. They also found an association between specific allele AGT (T235, rs699) with essential hypertension and preeclampsia. Angiotensin converting enzyme (ACE) along with AGT receptor 1 (AGTR1) were also found to have a role in the pathogenesis of the preeclampsia. Another candidate gene that link preeclampsia to the risk of hypertension is the T allele (C677T) of the methylenetetrahydrofolate reductase (MTHFR) gene [19–23].

To conclude, no single gene or chromosomal locus currently known can explain the pathogenesis of preeclampsia. This indicates that preeclampsia is a polygenic disorder, and it reflects an integrated pathophysiological process of insufficient adaptation, not only in the placenta, but also in other tissues and organs. On the other hand, the geographical distribution of candidate genes and loci in association with the pathogenesis of preeclampsia may reflect the interaction between the different environments and the gene pool of populations.

6. Adaptive polymorphisms of hypoxia genes

Here, we discuss some of the known genetic polymorphisms that influence maternal vascular adaptation in normal pregnancy and preeclampsia, high-altitude adaptation, and adaptive variants in healthy exercise. These genetic changes affect the protein activity and production, and can be set as early predictive markers for adaptation.

6.1 Endothelial nitric oxide synthase (eNOS): (rs1799983, G894T, Glu298Asp)

Healthy pregnancy is associated with enhanced endothelium-dependent vasodilation in the brachial artery, a response mediated by NO. These changes are thought to be an important physiological adaptation that accommodates the increased circulating blood volume and cardiac output during pregnancy. A common polymorphism of the eNOS gene is G894T in the mature protein that has been associated with the differences in endothelium-dependent dilation at 12-week gestation. There are several reports on the association between eNOS 894T allele polymorphism and PE susceptibility. They also provide a potential mechanism linking eNOS polymorphism with the prediction of cardiovascular disorders and pulmonary edema in which NO bioactivity is impaired [24–26].

In high-altitude adaptation, previous studies showed that the eNOS G894T polymorphism contributed to physiology and pathophysiology of humans at high altitude by regulating the production of NO. The 894G allele carriers and GG genotype might be a beneficial factor for HA adaptation through enhancing the level of NO, and 894T allele and heterozygous G/T of the 894G/T variant are associated with the susceptibility to high-altitude pulmonary edema (HAPE) at Qinghai-Tibet. In acclimatization to high altitude, NO levels increase dramatically above the baseline levels, while visitors ill with high-altitude pulmonary edema at the time of the study or in the past, have NO levels were lower than those of their healthy counterparts. Highland indigenous populations like Tibetans have high NO levels in the lung, plasma, and red blood cells that were at least double the levels that can be found in other populations regardless of altitude. With respect to NOS3 G894T and its relation to athletic performance or status, the over-representation of the GG genotype and G allele in all athletes suggests that the G894 allele may favor many types of sports [27, 28]. This supports the adaptive function of 894G allele and genotype.

Probably adaptive: 894G allele; less adaptive: 894 T allele

6.2 Angiotensin converting enzyme (ACE): (rs4646994, ACEI/D)

Circulating angiotensin I-converting enzyme (ACE) exerts a tonic regulatory function in circulatory homeostasis, through the synthesis of vasoconstrictor angiotensin II. ACE I/D (insertion/deletion) polymorphism is associated with ACE level. The presence (insertion, I allele) rather than the absence (deletion, D allele) of a287 bp Alu sequence insertion fragment is associated with lower serum and tissue ACE activity and thus lower angiotensin II production. The D allele of the ACE I/D polymorphism along with higher ACE levels were over-represented in Han Chinese who was afflicted with AMS. On ascent to extreme altitudes, the I allele of the ACEI/D polymorphism may tend to have more sufficient/efficient acclimatization and consequently have less risk of developing AMS. It was hypothesized that the pioneer lowlanders who migrated to high altitude might have the I-related genotypes (the II or ID genotype) as an "inner predisposition" to overcome altitude illnesses during migration and adaptation and finally was able to settle at high altitude permanently. However, some evidence shows that they may gain their adaptation through the long period of settlement. Along with elite mountaineers, the I allele has been associated with some aspects of endurance performance in Marathon runners, rowers, cyclists, handball players, and others in different population. In the prediction of the disease, it was shown that the ACE D allele leads to increased expression of plasminogen activator inhibitor-1 (PAI-1), which can increase the risk of preeclampsia and thrombotic events and enhances the production of angiotensin II from angiotensin I [29, 30].

Probably adaptive: ACE I allele; less adaptive: ACE D allele

6.3 Vascular endothelial growth factor (VEGFA): (rs3025039, C 936T)

Vascular endothelial growth factor (VEGF) is a major angiogenic factor that acts as a regulator of endothelial cell proliferation and vascular permeability. VEGF has been shown to be markedly up-regulated in hypoxic conditions. A common polymorphism of VEGFA is 936 C>T (rs3025039). The carriers of the 936T allele have lower VEGF plasma level by one-third of non-carriers. In a comparison between two groups of lowlanders on ascent to high altitude; those with 936T allele have a decreased risk of acute mountain sickness. In acute exercise, VEGF levels increases in sedentary individuals "less adaptive," whereas exercise adaptation attenuates VEGF gene expression in human skeletal muscle in trained "well adaptive" individuals. Both findings appear to be related in preeclamptic women, where the increased VEGF level is accompanied by the C allele of VEGFA. Thus, it is possible that the T allele associates with the maintenance of normal pregnancy and may confer a protective effect against the development of preeclampsia and is consistent with the concept of having the T allele and low VEGF levels among women with normal, uncomplicated pregnancies [31].

Probably adaptive: 936T allele; less adaptive: 936 C allele

6.4 HIF-2α/EPAS-1: high-altitude adaptive gene

It was recently shown that the gene encoding HIF-2α/EPAS-1 represents a key mutated gene in the adaptation of Tibetan populations at high altitudes. Although it is highly similar to HIF-1 and has the potential to bind and mediate many of the same genes as HIF-1, its biological actions in response to hypoxia are distinct from those of HIF-1. By now, several of these HIF-2 mediated processes have been implicated in the human response to high-altitude exposure including erythropoiesis, iron homeostasis, metabolism, and vascular permeability, which are perturbed in preeclampsia. HGB-decreasing allele of EPAS1 is under very strong positive selection in Tibetans and is strongly associated with Hb, red cell count, and hematocrit. Although there is no association between HIF-2α/EPAS-1 polymorphisms and preeclampsia in the literature, few studies found up-regulated expression of HIF-2α in preeclampsia. In earlier work, we discussed the association between EPAS1 polymorphisms and preeclampsia. Based on the strong positive association signal of adaptation in Tibetans, I emphasized on the role of EPAS1 in preeclampsia, and suggest and for the first time that the mutated EPAS1, has to be considered as a major player for placental adaptation in normal pregnancy and preeclampsia.

Further experimental studies are needed to confirm the biological function of EPAS-1 in normal pregnancy [3, 32–34].

6.5 Methylenetetrahydrofolate reductase (MTHFR) (rs1801133, A222 V, C677T)

The effects of MTHFR on preeclampsia are of great interest to researchers in the field. MTHFR plays a key role in homocysteine metabolism. Tibetans have an increased frequency of the homocysteine-decreasing allele of rs1801133 at the MTHFR locus more than other individuals from Eastern Asian ancestry. The homocysteine level in Tibetans is even lower than in Han, who lives at the same highlands of Tibet's but for shorter period. This renders them to be less adaptive compared to Tibetans. On the other hand, several studies found significant association at this locus with PE. The gene promoter of MTHFR is found to be hypermethylated in preeclamptic women, and this results in a high level of homocysteine. The same can be found in high-altitude sickness as a result of mal adaptation [35, 36].

7. Adaptive or less adaptive

Looking for adaptive variants is the "half-full" interpretation for the prediction of a multiple disorder like preeclampsia. The genetic scan can include adaptive genes and polymorphisms, their functional importance, i.e., effect on enzyme activity and production, their protective effect, i.e., protective from/at risk of cardiovascular disorders, pulmonary edema, thrombosis, thrombophilia, retinopathy, etc.

Earlier predictive markers for preeclampsia are believed to be in the first trimester, but it could be earlier even before the pregnancy period. Exercise stress test can be done to measure the levels of oxidative stress during and after the exercise to predict the possible response of the body. Allele and genotype frequencies of adaptive variants before the pregnancy, gene expression during and after the exercise can also be studied. In short, women who are less adaptive in their exercise have the potentials to develop preeclampsia. The same in high-altitude adaptation, women who suffer on ascent to high altitude are more likely to be preeclamptic.

"Adaptive or less adaptive" can be simply the final result of genetic tests that predict the disease, recurrence, and possible complications. DNA analysis for potential genetic markers may serve to screen for the risks of preeclampsia/eclampsia and other adverse pregnancy outcomes. Those with positive adaptive status are considered to be at decreased risk of developing preeclampsia. Certain genetic polymorphisms are attributed with certain adverse pregnancy outcomes.

8. Ischemic reperfusion stress: adaptation or insult

In 1964, Martin et al. show that maternal blood flow of spiral arteries in the intervillous space is intermittent in all normal pregnancies, and they wondered if this intermittency is a mechanism for regulating maternal placental blood flow. In preeclampsia, it is believed that the process of intermittent placental perfusion (ischemic/reperfusion) secondary to deficient trophoblast invasion is a key intermediary step in the pathogenesis of preeclampsia.[37, 38].

However, the process of ischemia and reperfusion is well known to be used in clinical settings in the area of coronary heart diseases to protect the heart from the harmful effects of subsequent, prolonged ischemia by the exposure of tissues to certain degrees of intermittent periods of hypoxia and reoxygenation. The process termed ischemic preconditioning has been demonstrated in patients with cardiovascular disease as well as in many other organs. The process, termed ischemic preconditioning, has been demonstrated in patients with cardiovascular disease as well as in many other organs. Recent evidence suggests that there are actually two distinct types of protection afforded by preconditioning, acute and delayed preconditioning. The protective effects of acute preconditioning are protein synthesis independent in short intervals, while the effects of delayed preconditioning require protein synthesis in tissues subjected to prolonged ischemia. Delayed preconditioning appears to be an adaptation response that is dependent on altered gene expression as well as the synthesis of new proteins, including NO pathway.

It has been postulated that hypoxic preconditioning might occur normally in placentae that develop at high altitude. Laboring placentae at 3100 m have little or no oxidative stress at the time of delivery, suggesting greater resistance to ischemia-reperfusion. Unlike pregnancies at sea level subjected to labor display evidence of oxidative stress. In fact, exercise can be considered as a form of remote ischemic conditioning, in which the stimulus is distant from the organ being protected. Remote ischemic conditioning has been termed "exercise in a device," especially suited for patients who are unable or unwilling to work out [39–41].

The question is can we consider the intermittency of maternal blood flow as a regulatory mechanism for natural hypoxic preconditioning that can occur in placentae from high altitude, and can it be the answer for the earlier question from the 1960s.

8.1 Genetics and ischemic preconditioning

Ischemic preconditioning reprograms the response to ischemic injury via transcriptional changes that resemble evolutionarily conserved responses to decreased blood flow and oxygen availability. The response to ischemia alters gene expression and induces cellular adaptations and hypoxia tolerance. One of the regulatory mechanisms is the genetic reprogramming through microRNAs. MiRNA-144 and -21 have been associated with ischemic preconditioning and normal pregnancy, and can be considered as adaptive miRNAs.

MicroRNA-144 is a circulating effector of remote ischemic preconditioning. Systemic release of microRNA-144 plays a pivotal role in inducing early and delayed cardioprotection with improved functional recovery and reduction in infarct size. Comparably, miRNA-144 was down-regulated in severe preeclampsia during the early stages of pregnancy, which supports the maladaptive nature of the disease.

***MicroRNA*-21** stimulates angiogenesis by inducing VEGF production. MiRNA-21 expression is required for local and remote ischemic preconditioning in multiple organ protection, including kidneys, heart, liver, and lungs. In sport genomics, several studies support the protective role of miRNA-21 as an important regulator of exercise adaptation and in the protection of many disorders including cardiovascular disorders. In normal pregnancy, miR-21 has been shown to enhance trophoblast proliferation and invasion via modulating the nodal signaling pathway, and involve in angiogenesis process positive regulator of VEGF-A and HIF-1α. Yet, the persistent of miRNA-21 angiogenic signal can be deleterious [42–46].

9. Structural adaptations of the placenta

The prominent histological changes represent the structural adaptations for placental ischemia, which creates a hostile environment for the preeclamptic placentae. A number of these histopathological changes have been described; namely placental infarcts, increased syncytial knots, hypovascularity of the villi, increased cytotrophoblastic proliferation, thickening of the sub-trophoblastic basement membrane, obliterated enlarged endothelial cells in the fetal capillaries, and atherosis of the spiral arteries in the placental bed. The volume of the intervillous space and the terminal villi are also decreased in proportion to the degree of preeclampsia. Some of the histological features like syncytial knots, cytotrophoblastic proliferation, thickening of sub-trophoblastic basement membrane, and hypovascular villi were observed in the placentae of normotensive women in varying degrees yet within normal limits [47].

Placental infarcts are small yellowish-white deposits of fibrin (a fibrous protein) of the placenta caused by the inadequate blood supply. They occur normally in the placenta as pregnancy progresses, and account about 25–30% of term normal pregnancies. The fetus usually is not affected by infarction of the placenta, unless the process is extensive. However, infarcts are found in nearly all cases of moderate or severe PIH. They are strongly associated with pregnancy-induced hypertension (PIH) and with growth-restricted babies. Moreover, several studies have found a direct correlation between the degree of PIH and the amount of infarction of the placenta. At molecular levels, plasminogen activator inhibitors (PAI-1/PAI-2), which regulate fibrinolysis, could be responsible for the very high levels of fibrin deposition in the intervillous space and the placental infarction observed in these pregnancies. The hypofibrinolytic genotypes 4G/4G and A/A of the PAI-1 gene are associated with the occurrence of mild preeclampsia. The insertion/deletion PAI-1 4G/5G polymorphism (rs1799889) was also found to have a significant association with preeclampsia [48, 49].

Acute atherosis is characterized by subendothelial lipid-filled foam cells, fibrinoid necrosis, and perivascular lymphocytic infiltration. This lesion is generally confined to non-transformed spiral arteries and is frequently observed in patients with preeclampsia. In early-onset preeclamptic patients, the polymorphisms in the regulator of G protein signaling 2 gene (RGS2) 3′UTR (C1114G, rs4606) of CG or GG genotype is more frequent in decidual spiral arteries in women with acute atherosis (resembling early stage of atherosclerosis). PIA-1, as an important regulator within the fibrinolytic system, has also been shown to be a risk indicator for venous and arterial thrombosis [50, 51].

Retroplacental hematoma (placental abruption) is having bleeding behind the placenta. This happens when the placenta starts separating prematurely due to bleeding and instability of uteroplacental vessels. The maternal MTHFR C677T polymorphism was found to be a risk factor for placental abruption. This agrees with the association of hyperhomocysteinemia with placental abruption [52, 53].

Syncytial knots: For oxygen requirement, the syncytium depends on the maternal blood flow to the intervillous space through the uteroplacental circulation. Reduced uteroplacental blood flow in hypertension may result in hypoxic damage to the syncytium. The damaged syncytium stimulates syncytial nuclear proliferation leading to syncytial knots formation. In an attempt to replace the degenerated syncytium, the cytotrophoblast cells undergo proliferation. Increased numbers of syncytial knots have been reported in placentae of pregnancies complicated by preeclampsia, probably to be induced by hypoxia. Syncytins 1 and 2 genes play a crucial role in trophoblast fusion stage of syncytial knot formation [47, 54].

10. The cross talk between syncytiotrophoblast and other remote organs

Throughout pregnancy, the cross talk between the placenta and other parts of the body is mainly relying on messages released from the syncytium into the maternal circulation. There are extracellular vesicles often referred to as syncytiotrophoblast extracellular vesicles (STBEVs) due to their syncytiotrophoblast cell of origin. They are believed to play an important role both in normal and dysfunctional pregnancies. They are released in form of exosomes, microvesicles, and apoptotic bodies that carry many syncytiotrophoblast derived factors such as mRNA, miRNA, proteins, and lipids. This gives a potentially rich source of biomarkers in complications involving placental dysfunction [55, 56].

Vascular endothelial cells: In preeclampsia, there is an increased release of placental STBEVs into the maternal circulation. It has been suggested that release of factors from the placenta in response to ischemia results in endothelial dysfunction of the maternal circulation. As a result, an imbalance of anticoagulation and procoagulation forces is found in preeclampsia as increases in proteins of the coagulation cascade, proangiogenic and antiangiogenic imbalance resulting in high sflt-1 levels that inactivate VEGF function, increased adhesion cell molecules are also significantly elevated including VCAM-1, ICAM-1, and E-selectin. An example of angiogenic imbalance is the syncytial knots that are enriched with sFlt1 protein. At least 25% of the measurable sFlt1 in the third-trimester maternal plasma is bound to circulating placental microparticles. The free detached syncytial knots are loaded with sFlt1 protein and mRNA. These findings suggest that STBEVs may cause endothelial damage and contribute to the endothelial dysfunction [57].

Paranchymal organs: In general, the histological changes, mainly in eclamptic phase of preeclampsia, are hemorrhagic and thrombotic in nature. They are found in the main parenchymatous organs: liver, kidneys, placenta, brain, and adrenals. The liver lesions, when present, take the form of irregular, focal subcapsular, and intraparenchymal hemorrhages. On histologic examination, there are fibrin thrombi in the portal capillaries and foci of hemorrhagic necrosis. The kidney lesions are variable. The glomeruli show marked swelling of endothelial cells, amorphous dense deposits on the endothelial side of the basement membrane, and mesangial cell hyperplasia. Immunofluorescent studies show an abundance of fibrin in glomeruli. In advanced cases, fibrin thrombi are present in the glomeruli and capillaries of the cortex. If widespread and severe, these thrombi may produce complete destruction of the cortex in the pattern referred to as bilateral renal cortical necrosis. The brain may have gross or microscopic foci of hemorrhage along with small vessel thrombosis. Similar changes are often found in the heart and the anterior pituitary [58].

At molecular level, circulating STBEVs can directly affect these remote organs (**Figure 2**). An example of this is the STBEVs uptake by the primary human coronary artery endothelial cells and the transfer of placenta specific miRNAs from STBEVs inside these recipient cells. The transferred miRNAs were functional, causing a downregulation of specific target genes, including the PE associated gene fms related tyrosine kinase 1 (FLT1). This suggests the ability of the placenta for endothelial reprogramming that may underlay the increased risk of cardiovascular disease reported for women with preeclampsia later in life. In kidneys, renal ischemic preconditioning up-regulates the expression of microRNA-21 in serum extracellular vesicles of exosomes in kidney and remote organs. This results in decreased apoptosis and reduced proinflammatory cytokines production in multiple organs including kidneys, heart, liver, and lungs. Another example is the role of STBEVs in thrombi formation. STBEVs released from preeclamptic placenta exhibit increased procoagulant tissue factor activity. Tissue factor is the primary initiator of coagulation in vivo. The increased numbers of circulating STBEVs in the blood of women with preeclampsia, along with the greater expression of tissue factor on preeclampstic STBEVs would be expected to comprise a substantial intravascular pro-thrombotic stimulus. A majority of deep venous thrombosis

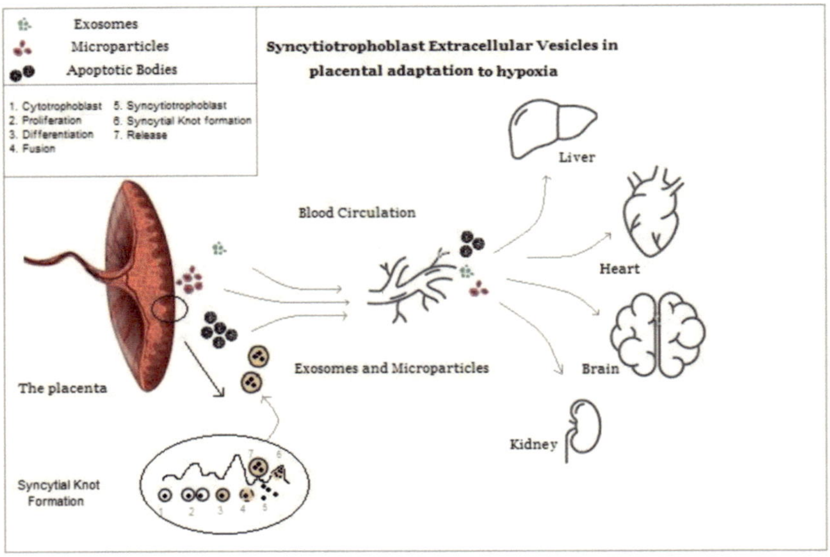

Figure 2.
The role of syncytiotrophoblast extracellular vesicles (STBEVs) in the cross talk between the placenta and other tissues and organs include exosomes, microvesicles, apoptotic bodies, and syncytial knots. Adequate blood flow from a limited number of EVs are shed from the placenta into the maternal circulation, while increased number of STBEVs are shed from preeclamptic placenta. The cargo of STBEVs including microRNAs, mRNAs, proteins, lipids, and glycans may be "planned" by the placenta. This cargo controls gene expression in vascular endothelial cells and other tissues and organs. STBEVs contents and deportations are controlled by the placental hypoxia. In preeclampsia, high levels of hypoxia lead to reduce syncytin-1 expression, and thus increased syncytial knots deportation [64].

occur within the valve pockets of deep venous valves that are exposed to "periods of stasis" and low oxygen levels, resembling the I/R oxidative stress. Venous valves have adapted to this phenomenon by expressing higher levels of anticoagulants thrombomodulin and endothelial cell protein C receptor, which are both decreased in preeclampsia [59–61].

To conclude, the high degree of concordance between placental lesions and gene expression across different subtypes of preeclampsia, reflects the importance of appropriate communication in successful pregnancy [62, 63].

11. Evolutionary steps: from preeclamptic cells, cancer to adaptive cells

Preeclamptic cells are genetically late compared to cancer cells, and this is probably the reason behind their protection from cancer. For example, angiogenesis are balanced in normal cells, and shift to the lift in preeclampsia and to the right in cancer cells and adaptive cells. The shift of preeclamptic cells from the left to the right can take longer time (**Figure 3**). Longer prospective studies show that preeclamptic women can lose their protective advantage by time, while adaptive individuals, according to the evolutionary steps, can show better protection than preeclamptic cells [65]. Normal cells can avoid cancer and jump to adaptive status by gradual adaptation or preconditioning. This is why normal multiple pregnancies are naturally protected from cancer and other oxidative stress disorders, due to their intermittent exposure to hypoxia that act as natural ischemic preconditioning. Accordingly, both preeclamptic cells and adaptive cells are protective against cancer, but for different reasons. In a different context, cancer cells, due to their high cellular turnout and high evolutionary rate, have a higher ability to gain mutations,

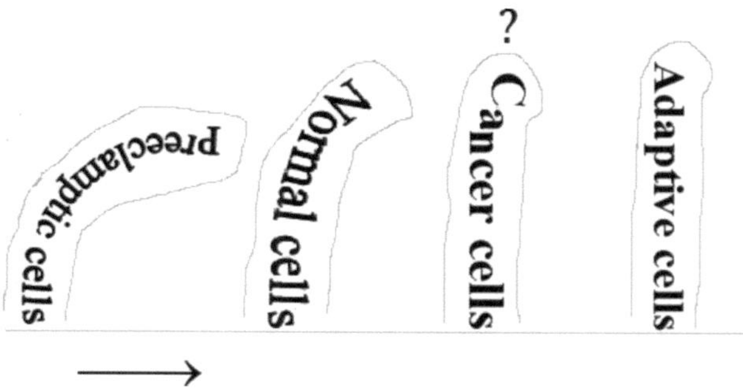

Figure 3.
Evolutionary steps from preeclamptic cells, normal cells, cancer cells, and adaptive cells.

and thus have a high probability for adaptive mutations. This can be used to study the protective function of adaptive variants in pregnancy and preeclampsia under different stressful conditions.

12. Conclusion

Future genetic studies are required for assaying additional adaptive variants near the candidate, HIF-targeted and -regulatory genes for testing functionality, and verify the existence of natural selection [9]. Such studies present a novel and relatively unexplored approach that enable the normal cells to adapt to their scarce microenvironment to the highest possible extent. No matter of the reasons that lead to preeclampsia, which are probably different, the advanced integrated biological system of genetic and epigenetic adaptive polymorphisms can "vaccinate" the body against the detrimental consequences and complications of the disease, and can reflect the ability of the body for survival and recovery. Methods of inducing natural adaptive mechanisms, like in ischemic preconditioning, has been attempted in clinical practice in the area of coronary heart disease in an attempt to limit the injury caused to the heart via ischemia and reperfusion injury. Such injury would occur when a patient has an acute myocardial infarction followed by reperfusion by either percutaneous coronary intervention or thrombolysis. Although, placental preconditioning was suggested to occur as an adaptive response to the hypobaric hypoxia at high altitudes, the area of placental preconditioning in clinical practice is yet to be explored. At molecular levels, adaptation to hypoxia can enhance the ability of the placenta to acquire genetic adaptive experience resulting in a stress relief, protection, and probably recovery in subsequent pregnancies. The messages released from the placenta into the maternal circulation transfer the genetic experience throughout the body. It can dramatically modify the histological picture in the placenta and other remote organs, and modulate the function of these organs.

Conflict of interest

The author declares no conflict of interest.

Author details

Sarah I.Y. Ahmed
Independent Researcher, Khartoum, Sudan

*Address all correspondence to: emailstosarah@gmail.com

References

[1] Darwin C. On The Origin of Species. 1861

[2] Dunwoodie SL. The role of hypoxia in development of the mammalian embryo. Developmental Cell. 2009;**17**(6):755-773. DOI: 10.1016/j.devcel.2009.11.008

[3] Ahmed SIY, Ibrahim ME, Khalil EAG. High altitude and pre-eclampsia: Adaptation or protection. Medical Hypotheses. 2017;**104**:128-132. DOI: 10.1016/j.mehy.2017.05.007

[4] Tal R. The role of hypoxia and hypoxia-inducible factor-1alpha in preeclampsia. Pathogenesis. 2012;**87**(October):1-8

[5] Rath G, Aggarwal R, Jawanjal P, Tripathi R, Batra A. HIF-1 alpha and placental growth factor in pregnancies complicated with preeclampsia: A qualitative and quantitative analysis. Journal of Clinical Laboratory Analysis. 2016;**30**:75-83

[6] Bianco-Miotto T, Buckberry S, Ricciardelli C, Leemaqz S, Khoda SM, Highet AR, et al. Hypoxia induced HIF-1/HIF-2 activity alters trophoblast transcriptional regulation and promotes invasion. European Journal of Cell Biology. 2015;**94**(12):589-602. DOI: 10.1016/j.ejcb.2015.10.004

[7] Rosario GX, Konno T, Soares MJ. Maternal hypoxia activates endovascular trophoblast cell invasion. Developmental Biology. 2009;**314**(2):362-375

[8] Julian CG. High altitude during pregnancy. Clinics in Chest Medicine. 2011;**32**(1):21-31. DOI: 10.1016/j.ccm.2010.10.008

[9] Moore LG, Shriver M, Bemis L, Hickler B, Wilson M, Brutsaert T, et al. Maternal adaptation to high-altitude pregnancy: An experiment of nature—A review. Placenta. 2004;**25**(Suppl. A): 60-71

[10] Tomar A, Malhotra S, Sarkar S. Polymorphism profiling of nine high altitude relevant candidate gene loci in acclimatized sojourners and adapted natives. BMC Genetics. 2015. DOI: 10.1186/s12863-015-0268-y

[11] Giannubilo SR, Landi B. Preeclampsia: What could happen in a subsequent pregnancy. Obstetrical & Gynecological Survey. 2014;**69**(12)

[12] Roberts JM, Hubel CA. The two stage model of preeclampsia: Variations on the theme. Placenta. 2010;**30**:1-12. Available from: http://istar.rwth-aachen.de/tiki-view_articles.php

[13] Galhardo RS, Hastings PJ, Rosenberg SM. Mutation as a stress response and the regulation of evolvability. Critical Reviews in Biochemistry and Molecular Biology. 2007;**42**:399-435

[14] Semsey S, Horvath P, Tuboly C, Krishna S, Hunziker A. Genetic flexibility of regulatory networks. Proceedings of the National Academy of Sciences. 2010;**107**(29):12998-13003

[15] Harrison GA, Humphrey KE, Jones N, Badenhop R, Guo G, Elakis G, et al. A genomewide linkage study of preeclampsia/eclampsia reveals evidence for a candidate region on 4q. American Journal of Human Genetics. 1997;**60**(5):1158-1167. Available from http://www.ncbi.nlm.nih.gov/pubmed/9150163

[16] Moses EK, Lade JA, Guo G, Wilton AN, Grehan M, Freed K, et al. A genome scan in families from Australia and New Zealand confirms the presence of a maternal susceptibility locus for pre-eclampsia, on chromosome 2.

American Journal of Human Genetics. 2000;**67**(6):1581-1585. Available from: https://www.sciencedirect.com/science/article/pii/S0002929707632285

[17] Laivuori H, Lahermo P, Ollikainen V, Widen E, Häivä-Mällinen L, Sundström H, et al. Susceptibility loci for preeclampsia on chromosomes 2p25 and 9p13 in Finnish families. American Journal of Human Genetics. 2003;**72**(1):168-177. Available from: http://www.ncbi.nlm.nih.gov/pubmed/12474145

[18] van Dijk M, Mulders J, Poutsma A, Könst AAM, Lachmeijer AMA, Dekker GA, et al. Maternal segregation of the Dutch preeclampsia locus at 10q22 with a new member of the winged helix gene family. Nature Genetics. 2005;**37**(5):514-519. Available from: http://www.ncbi.nlm.nih.gov/pubmed/15806103

[19] Yu CKH, Casas JP, Savvidou MD, Sahemey MK, Nicolaides KH, Hingorani AD. Endothelial nitric oxide synthase gene polymorphism (Glu298Asp) and development of pre-eclampsia: A case-control study and a meta-analysis. BMC Pregnancy Childbirth. 2006;**6**(7). Available from: http://www.ncbi.nlm.nih.gov/pubmed/16542455

[20] Fong FM, Sahemey MK, Hamedi G, Eyitayo R, Yates D, Kuan V, et al. Maternal genotype and severe preeclampsia: A HuGE review. American Journal of Epidemiology. 2014;**180**(4):335-345. Available from: https://academic.oup.com/aje/article-lookup/doi/10.1093/aje/kwu151

[21] Li X, Tan H, Zhou S, Hu S, Zhang T, Li Y, et al. Renin-angiotensin-aldosterone system gene polymorphisms in gestational hypertension and preeclampsia: A case-control gene-association study. Scientific Reports. 2016;**6**:38030. Available from: http://www.ncbi.nlm.nih.gov/pubmed/27910864

[22] Purkait P, Halder K, Thakur S, Ghosh Roy A, Raychaudhuri P, Bhattacharya S, et al. Association of angiotensinogen gene SNPs and haplotypes with risk of hypertension in eastern Indian population. Clinical Hypertension. 2017;**23**(1):12. Available from: http://www.ncbi.nlm.nih.gov/pubmed/28361007

[23] Zitouni H, Ben Ali Gannoum M, Raguema N, Maleh W, Zouari I, Faleh RE, et al. Contribution of angiotensinogen M235T and T174M gene variants and haplotypes to preeclampsia and its severity in (North African) Tunisians. Journal of the Renin-Angiotensin-Aldosterone System. 2018;**19**(1):147032031775392. Available from: http://journals.sagepub.com/doi/10.1177/1470320317753924

[24] Savvidou MD, Vallance PJT, Nicolaides KH, Hingorani AD. Endothelial nitric oxide synthase gene polymorphism and maternal vascular adaptation to pregnancy. Hypertension. 2001;**38**(6):1289-1293. Available from: http://www.ncbi.nlm.nih.gov/pubmed/11751705

[25] Droma Y, Hanaoka M, Ota M, Katsuyama Y, Koizumi T, Fujimoto K, et al. Positive association of the endothelial nitric oxide synthase gene polymorphisms with high-altitude pulmonary edema. Circulation. 2002;**106**(7):826-830

[26] Salimi S. The association of endothelial nitric oxide synthase gene polymorphisms and preeclampsia susceptibility. Gene, Cell and Tissue. 2015;**2**(1):1-2

[27] Sun YJ, Fang MW, Niu WQ, Li GP, Liu JL, Ding SQ, et al. Endothelial nitric oxide synthase gene polymorphisms associated with susceptibility to high altitude pulmonary edema in Chinese railway construction workers at Qinghai-Tibet over 4500 meters above

sea level. Chinese Medical Sciences Journal. 2010;**25**(4):215-221. DOI: 10.1016/S1001-9294(11)60005-9

[28] Eider J, Ficek K, Kaczmarczyk M, Maciejewska-Karłowska A, Sawczuk M, Cieszczyk P. Endothelial nitric oxide synthase g894t (rs1799983) gene polymorphism in polish athletes. Central European Journal of Biology. 2014;**9**(3):260-267

[29] Ahmetov II, Fedotovskaya ON. Current progress in sports genomics. In: Advances in Clinical Chemistry. 1st ed. Vol. 70. Elsevier Inc.; 2015. pp. 247-314. DOI: 10.1016/bs.acc.2015.03.003

[30] Fangfang W, Jie W, Yanlong Y, Xuefei L, Xuerong Z, Jie L, et al. Angiotensin-converting enzyme insertion/deletion (I/D) polymorphisms and recurrent pregnancy loss: a meta-analysis. Journal of Assisted Reproduction and Genetics. 2012;**29**(11):1167-1173

[31] Rogers MS, D'Amato RJ. Common polymorphisms in angiogenesis. Cold Spring Harbor Perspectives in Medicine. 2012;**2**(11):1-19

[32] Yang J, Jin Z, Chen J, Huang X, Li X, Liang Y, et al. Genetic signatures of high-altitude adaptation in Tibetans. Proceedings of the National Academy of Sciences of the United States of America. 2017;**114**(16):4189-4194

[33] Dai DM, Cao J, Yang HM, Sun HM, Su Y, Chen YY, et al. Hematocrit and plasma albumin levels difference may be a potential biomarker to discriminate preeclampsia and eclampsia in patients with hypertensive disorders of pregnancy. Clinica Chimica Acta. 2017;**464**(October 2015):218-222

[34] Sørensen S, Hoegh AM, Borup R, Nielsen FC, Hviid TVF. Gene expression profiling of placentas affected by pre-eclampsia. Journal of Biomedicine & Biotechnology. 2010;**2010**

[35] Zhao J, Wang Q, Zhang G, Luan Y, Yi J. Association between gene polymorphisms on chromosome 1 and susceptibility to pre-eclampsia: An updated meta-analysis. Medical Science Monitor. 2016;**22**:2202-2214

[36] Tang W, Wu X, Yang K, Liu J, Tang X, Sa Y, et al. Folate metabolism gene polymorphisms MTHFR C677T and A1298C and risk for preeclampsia: A meta-analysis. Journal of Assisted Reproduction and Genetics. 2015;**32**(5):797-805

[37] Hung TH, Burton GJ. Hypoxia and reoxygenation: A possible mechanism for placental oxidative stress in preeclampsia. Taiwanese Journal of Obstetrics & Gynecology. 2006;**45**(3):189-200. Available from. DOI: 10.1016/S1028-4559(09)60224-2

[38] Schoots MH, Gordijn SJ, Scherjon SA, van Goor H, Hillebrands JL. Oxidative stress in placental pathology. Placenta. 2018;**69**:153-161. DOI: 10.1016/j.placenta.2018.03.003

[39] Stokfisz K, Ledakowicz-Polak A, Zagorski M, Zielinska M. Ischaemic preconditioning—Current knowledge and potential future applications after 30 years of experience. Advances in Medical Sciences. 2017;**62**(2):307-316

[40] Murray AJ, Johns J, Beckey V, Tissot van Patot MC, Zwerdlinger L, Serkova NJ, et al. Human placental metabolic adaptation to chronic hypoxia, high altitude: Hypoxic preconditioning. American Journal of Physiology. Regulatory, Integrative and Comparative Physiology. 2009;**298**(1):R166-R172

[41] Stenzel-Poore MP, Stevens SL, Simon RP. Genomics of preconditioning. Stroke. 2004;**35**(11_suppl_1):2683-2686. DOI: 10.1161/01.STR.0000143735.89281.bb

[42] Li J, Rohailla S, Gelber N, Rutka J, Sabah N, Gladstone RA, et al.

MicroRNA-144 is a circulating effector of remote ischemic preconditioning. Basic Research in Cardiology. 2014;**109**(5):423. Available from: http://link.springer.com/10.1007/s00395-014-0423-z

[43] Barchitta M, Maugeri A, Quattrocchi A, Agrifoglio O, Agodi A. The role of miRNAs as biomarkers for pregnancy outcomes: A comprehensive review. International Journal of Genomics. 2017;**2017**:1-11. Available from: https://www.hindawi.com/journals/ijg/2017/8067972/

[44] Jia P, Wu X, Dai Y, Teng J, Fang Y, Hu J, et al. MicroRNA-21 is required for local and remote ischemic preconditioning in multiple organ protection against sepsis. Critical Care Medicine. 2017;**45**(7):e703-e710. Available from: http://www.ncbi.nlm.nih.gov/pubmed/28437377

[45] Bounds KR, Chiasson VL, Pan LJ, Gupta S, Chatterjee P. MicroRNAs: New players in the pathobiology of preeclampsia. Frontiers in Cardiovascular Medicine. 2017;**4**:60. Available from: http://www.ncbi.nlm.nih.gov/pubmed/28993808

[46] Silva GJJ, Bye A, El Azzouzi H, Wisløff U. MicroRNAs as important regulators of exercise adaptation. Progress in Cardiovascular Diseases. 2017;**60**(1):130-151. Available from: http://www.ncbi.nlm.nih.gov/pubmed/28666746

[47] Gunasena GA, Jayasundara D, Salgado SS, Wijesinghe P, Biyagama BRGDNK. The placenta in pre-eclampsia: Association of histology with umbilical artery Doppler velocimetry. Women's Health. 2017;**4**(4):90-94. Available from: http://medcraveonline.com/MOJWH/MOJWH-04-00092.php

[48] Fabbro D, D'Elia AV, Spizzo R, Driul L, Barillari G, Di Loreto C, et al. Association between plasminogen activator inhibitor 1 gene polymorphisms and preeclampsia. Gynecologic and Obstetric Investigation. 2003;**56**(1):17-22. Available from: http://www.ncbi.nlm.nih.gov/pubmed/12867763

[49] Zhao L, Bracken MB, DeWan AT, Chen S. Association between the SERPINE1 (PAI-1) 4G/5G insertion/deletion promoter polymorphism (rs1799889) and pre-eclampsia: A systematic review and meta-analysis. Mol Hum Reprod. 2013;**19**(3):136-143. Available from: https://academic.oup.com/molehr/article-lookup/doi/10.1093/molehr/gas056

[50] Kim YM, Chaemsaithong P, Romero R, Shaman M, Kim CJ, Kim J-S, et al. The frequency of acute atherosis in normal pregnancy and preterm labor, preeclampsia, small-for-gestational age, fetal death and midtrimester spontaneous abortion. Journal of Maternal-Fetal & Neonatal Medicine. 2015;**28**(17):2001-2009. Available from: http://www.ncbi.nlm.nih.gov/pubmed/25308204

[51] Kvehaugen AS, Melien Ø, Holmen OL, Laivuori H, Øian P, Andersgaard AB, et al. Single nucleotide polymorphisms in G protein signaling pathway genes in preeclampsia. Hypertension. 2013;**61**(3):655-661. Available from: https://www.ahajournals.org/doi/10.1161/HYPERTENSIONAHA.111.00331

[52] Nurk E, Tell GS, Refsum H, Ueland PM, Vollset SE. Associations between maternal methylenetetrahydrofolate reductase polymorphisms and adverse outcomes of pregnancy: The Hordaland Homocysteine Study. The American Journal of Medicine. 2004;**117**(1):26-31. Available from: http://www.ncbi.nlm.nih.gov/pubmed/15210385

[53] Ray J, Laskin C. Folic acid and homocyst(e)ine metabolic defects and the risk of placental abruption, pre-eclampsia and spontaneous

pregnancy loss: A systematic review. Placenta. 1999;**20**(7):519-529. Available from: http://www.ncbi.nlm.nih.gov/pubmed/10452905

[54] Vargas A, Toufaily C, LeBellego F, Rassart É, Lafond J, Barbeau B. Reduced expression of both syncytin 1 and syncytin 2 correlates with severity of preeclampsia. Reproductive Sciences. 2011;**18**(11):1085-1091. Available from: http://journals.sagepub.com/doi/10.1177/1933719111404608

[55] Tannetta D, Collett G, Vatish M, Redman C, Sargent I. Syncytiotrophoblast extracellular vesicles—Circulating biopsies reflecting placental health. Placenta. 2017;**52**:134-138. Available from: http://www.ncbi.nlm.nih.gov/pubmed/27899180

[56] Cronqvist T, Tannetta D, Mörgelin M, Belting M, Sargent I, Familari M, et al. Syncytiotrophoblast derived extracellular vesicles transfer functional placental miRNAs to primary human endothelial cells. Scientific Reports. 2017;**7**(1):4558. Available from: http://www.ncbi.nlm.nih.gov/pubmed/28676635

[57] Rajakumar A, Cerdeira AS, Rana S, Zsengeller Z, Edmunds L, Jeyabalan A, et al. Transcriptionally active syncytial aggregates in the maternal circulation may contribute to circulating soluble Fms-like tyrosine kinase 1 in preeclampsia. Hypertension. 2012;**59**(2):256-264. Available from: https://www.ahajournals.org/doi/10.1161/HYPERTENSIONAHA.111.182170

[58] Govan AD. The histology of eclamptic lesions. Journal of Clinical Pathology. Supplement (Royal College of Pathologists). 1976;**10**:63-69. Available from: http://www.ncbi.nlm.nih.gov/pubmed/1067270

[59] Shamshirsaz AA, Paidas M, Krikun G. Preeclampsia, hypoxia, thrombosis, and inflammation. Journal of Pregnancy. 2012;**2012**:374047. Available from: http://www.ncbi.nlm.nih.gov/pubmed/22175023

[60] Turner RJ, Bloemenkamp KWM, Bruijn JA, Baelde HJ. Loss of thrombomodulin in placental dysfunction in preeclampsia. Arteriosclerosis, Thrombosis, and Vascular Biology. 2016;**36**(4):728-735. Available from: http://www.ncbi.nlm.nih.gov/pubmed/26891741

[61] Zhu JM, He M, Huang L, Su YL, Li L, Li M. Expression and significance of EPCR in plasma and placenta of patients with early onset severe preeclampsia. Zhonghua Fu Chan Ke Za Zhi. 2016;**51**(9):678-682. Available from: http://www.ncbi.nlm.nih.gov/pubmed/27671049

[62] Benton SJ, Leavey K, Grynspan D, Cox BJ, Bainbridge SA. The clinical heterogeneity of preeclampsia is related to both placental gene expression and placental histopathology. American Journal of Obstetrics and Gynecology. 2018;**219**(6):604.e1-604.e25. Available from: http://www.ncbi.nlm.nih.gov/pubmed/30278173

[63] Escudero CA, Herlitz K, Troncoso F, Acurio J, Aguayo C, Roberts JM, et al. Role of extracellular vesicles and microRNAs on dysfunctional angiogenesis during preeclamptic pregnancies. Frontiers in Physiology. 2016;**7**:98. Available from: http://journal.frontiersin.org/Article/10.3389/fphys.2016.00098/abstract

[64] Roland CS, Hu J, Ren C-E, Chen H, Li J, Varvoutis MS, et al. Morphological changes of placental syncytium and their implications for the pathogenesis of preeclampsia. Cellular and Molecular Life Sciences. 2016;**73**(2):365-376. Available from: http://www.ncbi.nlm.nih.gov/pubmed/26496726

[65] Taylor A. Pre-eclampsia and the risk of cancer. BMJ. 2004;**328**:909-910

Chapter 4

Clinical, Biochemical, and Biophysical Markers of Angiogenesis in Preeclampsia

Osredkar Joško and Kumer Kristina

Abstract

Preeclampsia/eclampsia is described as a pregnancy-specific systemic disorder of unknown etiology and is a potentially life-threatening disease with symptoms related to a general vascular endothelial cell activation and dysfunction. Preeclampsia can be defined as a new onset of hypertension (>140/90 mmHg) after gestational week 20 together with significant proteinuria (300 mg/24 h). Preeclampsia has a complex pathophysiology, the primary cause likely being abnormal placentation. Angiogenic factors and biophysical markers may be combined for predicting preeclampsia. Various high-throughput techniques have evolved, thus allowing us simultaneous examination of thousands of genes (genomics), gene transcripts (transcriptomics), proteins (proteomics), metabolites (metabolomics), protein interaction (interactomics), and chromatin modifications (epigenomics) in single experiments, and the results suggest that the use of transcriptomic, proteomic, and metabolomic profiles may be predictive for preeclampsia.

Keywords: preeclampsia, biomarkers, sFlt-1, PlGF, sEndoglin

1. Classification and epidemiology of hypertension during pregnancy

Hypertension is the second most prevalent maternal complication worldwide after anemia in pregnancy, and it is associated with a significant morbidity and mortality of the mother and fetus. The American College of Obstetricians and Gynecologists Task Force on Hypertension in Pregnancy has modified the older classification of hypertension during pregnancy in only four categories: (1) preeclampsia-eclampsia, (2) chronic hypertension (of any cause), (3) chronic hypertension with superimposed preeclampsia, and (4) gestational hypertension (**Figure 1**). It has been suggested that an older category, "unclassified," be reintroduced or replaced by "suspected" or "presumptive" preeclampsia [1].

In 2017, the American College of Cardiology and American Heart Association (ACC/AHA) issued a clinical practice guideline on hypertension that reclassified the previous category of prehypertension into elevated BP (systolic BP 120–129 mmHg) and stage 1 hypertension (systolic BP 130–139 mmHg or diastolic BP 80–89 mmHg) [2]. However a rise of diastolic blood pressure over prepregnant levels (delta hypertension) rather than a rise above absolute value is also a significant predictive marker.

Severe features of preeclampsia (any of these findings):

A. Systolic blood pressure of 160 mmHg or higher or diastolic blood pressure of 110 mmHg or higher on two occasions at least 4 h apart

B. Thrombocytopenia

C. Impaired liver function as indicated by abnormally elevated liver enzymes

D. Progressive renal insufficiency

E. Pulmonary edema

F. New-onset cerebral or visual disturbances

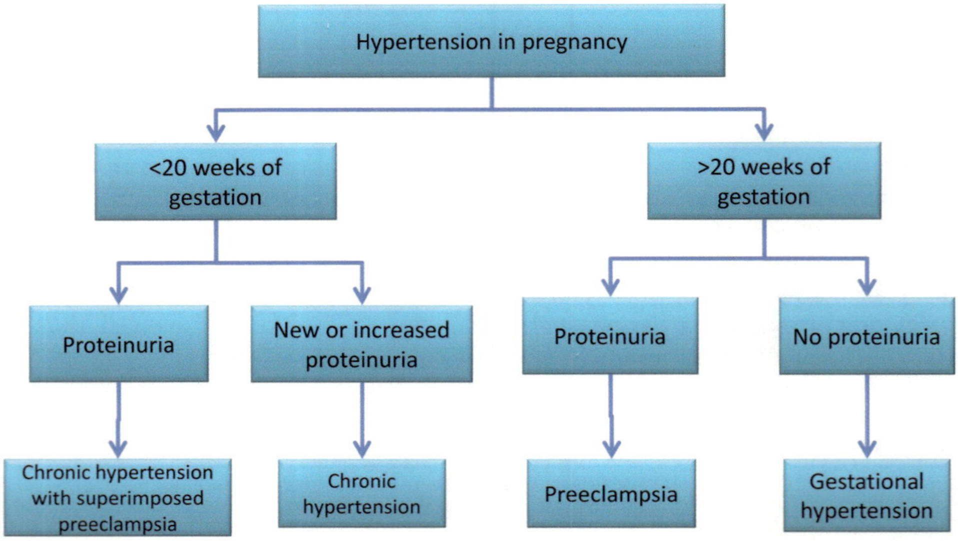

Figure 1.
Classification of hypertensive disorders in pregnancy.

2. Definition of preeclampsia

Preeclampsia/eclampsia is described as a pregnancy-specific systemic disorder of unknown etiology and is a potentially serious disease with symptoms related to a generalized vascular endothelial activation. The placenta seems to be a crucial component in the pathophysiology of the disease. Preeclampsia is a multisystemic disease characterized by the development of hypertension after 20 weeks of gestation, with the presence of proteinuria or, in its absence, of signs or symptoms indicative of target organ injury [3, 4].

Preeclampsia can be defined as a new onset of hypertension (>140/90 mmHg) after gestational week 20 together with significant proteinuria (300 mg/24 h) [5, 6]. Hypertension is considered mild until diastolic or systolic levels reach or exceed 110 and 160 mmHg, respectively. It is recommended that a diagnosis of hypertension requires at least two determinations at least 4 h apart. Proteinuria is diagnosed when 24-h excretion equals or exceeds 300 mg in 24 h or the ratio of measured protein to creatinine in a single-voided urine measures or exceeds 0.3 (each measured as mg/dL), termed the urinary protein/creatinine ratio [1]. The definitive treatment of preeclampsia is delivery to prevent development of maternal or fetal complications from disease progression. Timing of delivery is based upon gestational age, the severity of preeclampsia, and maternal and fetal condition.

3. Key elements of the pathophysiology

Precise causes of preeclampsia are still unknown, but contributors are impaired angiogenesis [7], systemic endothelial dysfunction [8], and decreased vascular compliance resulting in impaired accommodation of the volume expansion required for healthy gestation [9].

During normal pregnancy, the villous cytotrophoblast invades into the inner third of the myometrium, and spiral arteries are remodeled. The remodeling contains four steps: decidua-associated remodeling, the intraluminal appearance of migratory endovascular trophoblasts, their intramural incorporation and trophoblast-associated remodeling, and maternal reendothelialization.

Preeclampsia has a complex pathophysiology, the primary cause likely being abnormal placentation. Defective invasion of the spiral arteries by cytotrophoblast cells is observed during preeclampsia. Recent studies have shown that cytotrophoblast invasion of the uterus is actually a unique differentiation pathway in which the fetal cells adopt certain attributes of the maternal endothelium they normally replace. In preeclampsia, this differentiation process is defective [10].

In normal pregnancy the uterine arteries are resilient and elastic, and they lose their sensitivity to vasoconstrictors. In a preeclamptic pregnancy there is increased uterine arterial resistance and higher sensitivity to vasoconstrictors and thus chronic placental ischemia and oxidative stress. This chronic placental ischemia causes fetal complications, including fetal growth restriction (FGR) and intrauterine death. In parallel, oxidative stress induces release into the maternal circulation of substances such as free radicals, oxidized lipids, cytokines, and serum soluble vascular endothelial growth factor receptor 1 (sVEGFR-1/sFlt-1). These abnormalities are responsible for endothelial dysfunction [8] with vascular hyperpermeability, thrombophilia, and hypertension, so as to compensate for the decreased blood flow in the uterine arteries due to peripheral vasoconstriction. Endothelial dysfunction is responsible for the clinical signs observed in the mother, i.e., impairment of the hepatic endothelium contributing to onset of the HELLP (hemolysis, elevated liver enzymes, and low platelet count) syndrome, impairment of the cerebral endothelium inducing cerebral edema or posterior

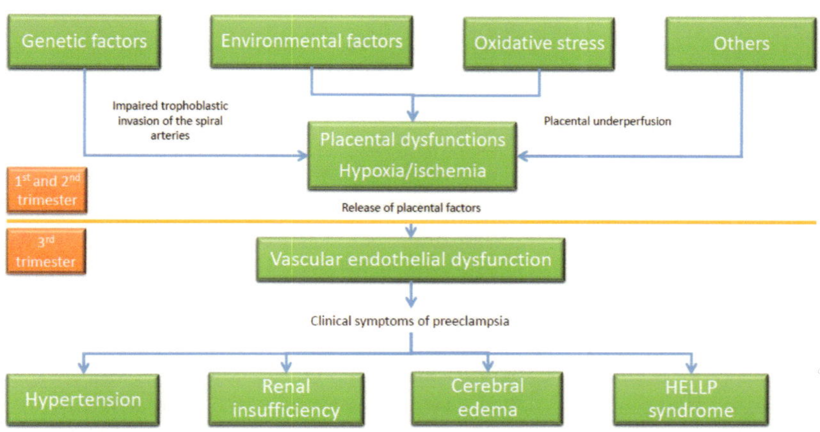

Figure 2.
Pathogenesis of preeclampsia.

reversible encephalopathy syndrome (PRES), refractory neurological disorders, or even eclampsia. In kidney, the depletion of vascular endothelial growth factor (VEGF) in the podocytes leads to endotheliosis, and these block the slit diaphragms in the basement membrane, exacerbating the already decreased glomerular filtration and causing proteinuria. Finally, endothelial dysfunction promotes microangiopathic hemolytic anemia, and vascular hyperpermeability associated with low serum albumin causes edema, particularly in the lower limbs or lungs. The crucial issue to understand is that the prime mover of preeclampsia is abnormal placentation [11] [**Figure 2**].

4. Symptoms

Preeclampsia sometimes develops without any symptoms. High blood pressure may develop slowly, or it may have a sudden onset. Monitoring of blood pressure is an important part of prenatal care because the first sign of preeclampsia is commonly a rise in blood pressure. Blood pressure that exceeds 140/90 mmHg—documented on two occasions, at least 4 h apart—is considered abnormal.

Other signs and symptoms of preeclampsia may include:

- Excess protein in urine (proteinuria)
- Severe headaches
- Vision changes include sensations of flashing lights, light sensitivity, blurry vision, or spots
- Upper abdominal pain, usually under ribs on the right side
- Nausea or vomiting
- Decreased urine output
- Decreased levels of platelets in the blood (thrombocytopenia)
- Impaired liver function
- Shortness of breath and anxiety
- Sudden weight gain
- Swelling (edema)

Many of these symptoms also occur in normal pregnancies, so they are not considered reliable signs of preeclampsia though they will alert the obstetrician.

The International Society of Study of Hypertension in Pregnancy (ISSHP) recently suggested that a clinical diagnosis is made even in the absence of proteinuria if organ-specific signs or symptoms are present with new onset of hypertension [12].

Hemolysis, abnormal elevation of liver enzymes levels, and low platelet count occur together as the HELLP syndrome [13]. HELLP syndrome is a severe variant of preeclampsia that occurs in 5% of cases and can progress rapidly to a life-threatening condition [14]. The presence of seizures in preeclampsia is eclampsia and is another complication during pregnancy and at delivery. In **Table 1**, diagnostic criteria are summarized.

Blood pressure
• Greater than or equal to 140 mm Hg systolic or greater than or equal to 90 mm Hg diastolic on two occasions at least 4 h apart after 20 weeks of gestation in a woman with a previously normal blood pressure
• Greater than or equal to 160 mm Hg systolic or greater than or equal to 110 mm Hg diastolic; hypertension can be confirmed within a short interval (minutes) to facilitate timely antihypertensive therapy
and
Proteinuria
• Greater than or equal to 300 mg per 24 h urine collection (or this amount extrapolated from a timed collection)
or
• Protein/creatinine ratio greater than or equal to 0.3*
• Dipstick reading of 1+ (used only if other quantitative methods not available)
Or in the absence of proteinuria, new-onset hypertension with the new onset of any of the following:
Thrombocytopenia
• Platelet count less than 100,000/μl
Renal insufficiency
• Serum creatinine concentrations greater than 1.1 mg/dL or a doubling of the serum creatinine concentration (normal levels in pregnancy are 0.8 mg/dL) in the absence of other renal disease
Impaired liver function
• Elevated blood concentrations of liver transaminases to twice normal concentration
Pulmonary edema
Cerebral or visual symptoms

Each measured as mg/dL.

Table 1.
Diagnostic criteria for preeclampsia by ACOG.

5. Risk factors of preeclampsia

Risk factors include health conditions, lifestyle, and family history that can increase the risk for high blood pressure.

Some of the risk factors for high blood pressure cannot be controlled, such as age or family history. But we can take steps to lower our risk by changing the factors we can control.

Some medical conditions can raise the risk for high blood pressure. If one of these risks is present, the pregnant women can take steps to control it and lower the risk. However preeclampsia cannot be prevented, but the complications of preeclampsia can be prevented.

ACOG recommendation, any risk factor [1]	NICE guidelines, one high risk or two moderate risk factors [15]
Risk factors	**High risk factors**
Nulliparity	Hypertensive disease in previous pregnancy
Age > 40 years	Chronic kidney disease
BMI > 30 kg/m^2	Diabetes mellitus
Family history of PE	Chronic hypertension
History of previous pregnancy with PE	Autoimmune disease

ACOG recommendation, any risk factor [1]	NICE guidelines, one high risk or two moderate risk factors [15]
Conception by in vitro fertilization	
Chronic hypertension	**Moderate risk factors**
Chronic renal disease	Nulliparity
Diabetes mellitus	Age > 40 years
Systemic lupus erythematosus	Interpregnancy interval > 10 years
Thrombophilia	BMI at first visit > 35 kg/m^2
	Chronic hypertension

ACOG, American College of Obstetricians and Gynecologists; NICE, National Institute of Clinical Excellence; PE, preeclampsia

Table 2.
Risk factors for preeclampsia by ACOG and NICE recommendations.

Preeclampsia develops only as a complication of pregnancy. Risk factors are presented in **Table 2** together with data of increased risk for some items [15].

The National Institute for Health and Care Excellence (NICE) recommends that women with high and more than one of the moderate risk factors for preeclampsia should be advised to take aspirin from 12 weeks gestation [16].

6. Biochemical markers

The role of biomarkers in preeclampsia diagnosis is becoming increasingly important. A literature review gives us a range of biomarkers that have proved to be sufficiently specific and sensitive to be classified as potential biomarkers (**Figure 3**). The most researched with data on specificity and sensitivity are given in **Table 3**. A good biomarker would be one, which may have the potential of identifying women earlier in their disease course. There have been also many studies investigating multiple-marker algorithms for predicting preeclampsia.

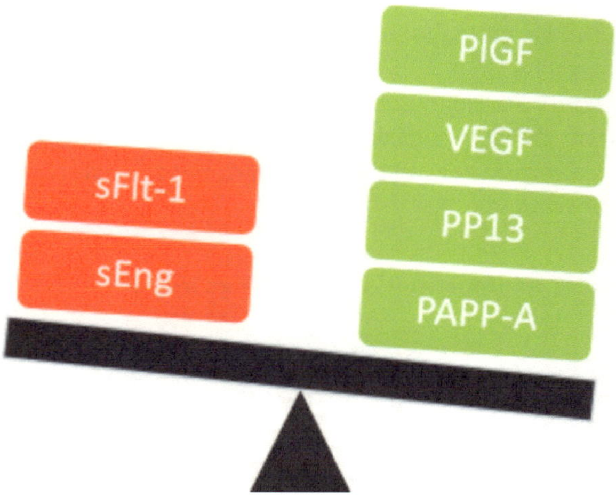

Figure 3.
Biochemical markers in preeclampsia. sFlt-1, soluble fms-like tyrosine kinase 1; PlGF, placental growth factor; sEng, soluble endoglin; PP13, placental protein 13; PAPP-A, pregnancy-associated plasma protein A.

Biomarker	Sensitivity	Specificity
sFlt-1	26–73.1%	88.5–100%
PlGF	64.1%	89.5%
sFlt-1/ PlGF	78%	84%
sEng	18–85%	69–84.6%
PP13	79–100%	80–90%
PAPP-A 1st trimester	49.7–69.7%	68.6–85.7%
NGAL	97.89%	93.55%
Insulin resistance	73%	85%
SHBG	85%	37.7%
Inhibin A and activin A	87%	80%
Copeptin 1st trimester	88%	81%
Uterine artery Doppler	Positive likelihood ratio 9:1	
Podocytes	38–100%	70–100%

sFlT-1, soluble fms-like tyrosine kinase 1; NGAL, neutrophil gelatinase-associated lipocalin; PAPP, pregnancy-associated plasma protein; PP, placental protein; sEng, soluble endoglin; SHBG, sex hormone-binding globulin

Table 3.
Biomarker test characteristics for prediction.

6.1 Soluble fms-like tyrosine kinase 1 (sFlt-1)

Soluble Flt-1 is an anti-angiogenic form of VEGF receptor 1. sFlt-1 acts as a potent scavenger of VEGF and PlGF (**Figure 4**), thus preventing their interaction with endothelial receptors on the cell surface, and subsequently induces endothelial dysfunction. Elevated concentration of sFlt-1 has been as early as 5 weeks before the diagnosis of preeclampsia and correlates with severity of disease [17, 18]. Some other studies also support this sFlt-1 role in the pathogenesis of preeclampsia [19–21].

6.2 Placental growth factor

Placental growth factor (PlGF) is a prominent angiogenic factor in the development of the placental vascular system [22, 23]. During normal pregnancy, PlGF can

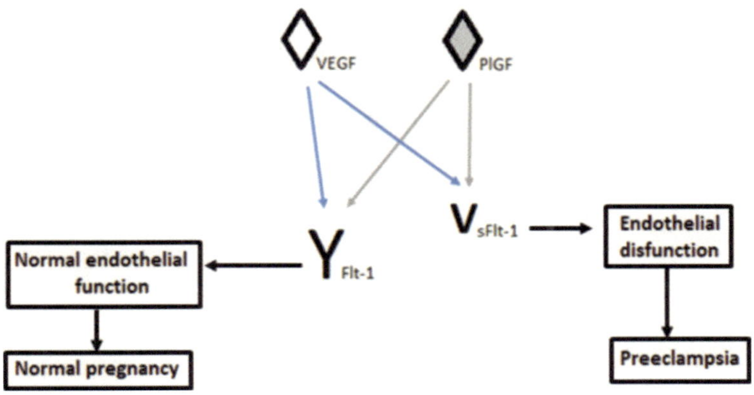

Figure 4.
Circulating sFlt-1 in the maternal blood leads to a net decrease in PlGF and VEGF in the vasculature, which are necessary for normal placental angiogenesis. In PE angiogenic balance is disturbed and may result in endothelial dysfunction.

be detected in the maternal circulation from 8 weeks gestation, reaching a maximal concentration toward the end of second trimester and declining thereafter until delivery [24]. In line with its pro-angiogenic function, reduced levels of PlGF were found in preeclampsia [18, 25, 26].

The commercial kits available for determination of PlGF are mostly using sandwich enzyme-linked immunosorbent assay (ELISA) (Roche Diagnostics International, Thermo Fisher Scientific, IBL International, Abcam) or fluoroimmunometricassay (PerkinElmer). In a multicenter, prospective study PROGNOSIS the Elecsys (Roche) sFlt-1/PlGF ratio proved to be a helpful tool in enabling clinicians to rule out the occurrence of preeclampsia for 1 week at cutoff of 38 or lower in women in whom the syndrome is suspected clinically. A ratio more than 38 indicates an increased risk of developing preeclampsia in the next 4 weeks [27].

6.3 sEndoglin

Endoglin (Eng) is a type I membrane glycoprotein localized to the cell membrane where it constitutes the transmembrane co-receptor for TGF beta receptor complex (TGF-β1 and TGF-β3) [28]. Circulating sEng was found to be high in preeclamptic women even prior to the disease manifestations correlating with disease severity and falls after delivery [17, 29], making it a reliable predictor of patients destined to develop severe early-onset preeclampsia [30].

Research has shown that near the time of delivery there is a rise in anti-angiogenic factors including [31, 32] soluble endoglin (sEng) [33], a drop in the pro-angiogenic placental growth factor (PlGF) [17], and slight changes in the vascular endothelial growth factor (VEGF) [34]. These have been associated with increases in the anti-angiogenic sFlt-1/PlGF ratio [35] and a decrease in the pro-angiogenic PlGF/(sFlt-1 + sEng) ratio [36, 37].

Other studies have reported increases in inhibin A [38] and placental protein 13 (PP13) [39] near delivery. The elevated tumor necrosis factor alpha (TNFα) has been detected in preterm delivery [40] and also in FGR [41].

6.4 Placental protein 13 (PP13)

PP13 is a member of the galectin family, predominantly expressed by the syncytiotrophoblast, during placental vascular development [42, 43]. Serum concentrations of PP13 are significantly lower in women who later develop preeclampsia, FGR, and preterm birth [39, 44]. Combining first trimester PP13 with other parameters may further improve predictive performance.

6.5 Pregnancy-associated plasma protein A (PAPP-A)

PAPP-A is a peptidase produced by syncytiotrophoblast with hydrolytic activity for insulin-like growth factor-binding proteins [45, 46]. Decreased levels of PAPP-A in the first trimester have been associated with increased risk of preeclampsia [47], not a good predictor of late-onset preeclampsia [48].

6.6 Free fetal nucleic acids

The examination of fetal cells, specifically erythroblasts, and of cell-free fetal DNA from the blood of pregnant women is a subject of intense research, with the aim of developing new risk-free methods for prenatal diagnosis [49, 50]. In preeclamptic pregnancies [51], cell-free fetal DNA is elevated long before the

Biomarker	The characteristics for prediction (95% Cl)
PAPP-A	Sensitivity 0.30 (0.29–0.32) Specificity 0.92 (0.92–0.92)
Inhibin A	Sensitivity 0.32 (0.25–0.39) Specificity 0.90 (0.89–0.91)
PP13	Sensitivity 0.37 (0.33–0.41) Specificity 0.88 (0.87–0.89)
PlGF	Sensitivity 0.65 (0.63–0.67) Specificity 0.89 (0.89–0.89)

Table 4.
The pooled sensitivity and specificity of the separate meta-analyses for some biomarkers.

clinical onset of the disease [52, 53]. Total free DNA has also been used and has been reported to be increased in women who subsequently develop preeclampsia [54].

New methods based on immunodiagnostics that measure the level of biomarkers as well as sonographic devices that measure the uterine artery blood flow have emerged as promising avenues that can lead to more accurate differential diagnoses.

6.7 Biophysical markers

Biophysical markers have also been developed to evaluate blood flow through the uterine arteries to the placenta. In the case of preeclampsia, an abnormal placentation results in decreased penetration of maternal spiral arteries in the junctional zone myometrium by cytotrophoblast cells. The consequence is that high blood flow and low-resistance vessels do not occur. Doppler ultrasonography has been evaluated as a potential predictive test for preeclampsia. Parameters such as the resistance index to the flow (RI), the average pulsatility index (PI), and the peak systolic flow (PSF) have been identified [55–58, 76].

6.8 Combination of tests

Angiogenic factors and biophysical markers may be combined for predicting preeclampsia. The combinations which give us best results are biochemical markers sFlt-1 and PlGF with Doppler [59, 60] and additional sEng [36] or PP13 [36, 61–63] and PAPP-A [63–66]. The pooled sensitivity of all single biomarkers for PE was 0.40 (95% Cl 0.39–0.41) at a false-positive rate of 10%. The area under the summary of receiver operating characteristic curve (SROC) was 0.786. The pooled sensitivity and specificity of the separate meta-analyses for some biomarkers are shown in **Table 4**. Wu et al. in their study got a pooled sensitivity of 0.91 (95% Cl: 0.90–0.91) and SROC of 0.893 for a combination of clinical characteristics, biomarkers, and Doppler pulsatility indexes [67].

7. Novel methods of diagnosis

Nowadays, various high-throughput techniques have evolved, thus allowing us simultaneous examination of thousands of genes (genomics), gene transcripts (transcriptomics), proteins (proteomics), metabolites (metabolomics), protein interaction (interactomics), and chromatin modifications (epigenomics) in single experiments.

mRNA-circulating placenta-specific mRNA in serum from preeclamptic women might be useful for the prediction of preeclampsia. In this study inhibin A, p-selectin, and VEGF receptor mRNA values were higher in preeclampsia, whereas human placental lactogen, KISS-1, and plasminogen activator type 1 were lower, both compared to normotensive controls [68]. Similar results were reported from some other studies also [69, 70], where circulating cells of fetal/placental origin were a source of mRNA. mRNAs were increased in women with preeclampsia, and there was a direct correlation between expression levels and the severity of the disease.

Protein, a functional product of gene expression can be measured. A set of differently expressed proteins which are involved in lipid metabolism, coagulation, complement regulation, extracellular matrix remodeling, protease inhibitor activity, and acute phase responses can be measured. A different pattern of proteins between the group of women who subsequently developed preeclampsia on one side and without preeclampsia on the other side [71] was reported. It is also reported that women with severe preeclampsia have a unique urine proteomic pattern [72] and that this proteomic profile appeared more than 10 weeks before the clinical manifestations, and this distinguished preeclampsia from other hypertensive or proteinuric disorders in pregnancy [73].

Some studies revealed that metabolomic strategies might be appropriate for investigating the metabolic function of trophoblast or placental tissue, and it was found that preeclamptic pregnancies have a different metabolomic profile when compared to normal pregnancies [74, 75].

These novel technologies in preeclampsia appear quite promising. The number of studies is growing, and the results suggest that the use of transcriptomic, proteomic, and metabolomic profiles may be predictive for preeclampsia. These techniques open new possibilities to find a new set of biomarkers for preeclampsia. Future studies are needed, with the collaborative efforts of bioinformatics, biostatistics, researchers, and clinicians.

Key points

- **A.** Preeclampsia is a pregnancy-specific hypertensive disorder with or without proteinuria that occurs after 20 weeks of gestation in a previously normotensive woman. In the absence of proteinuria, the diagnosis can still be made if new-onset hypertension is accompanied by signs or symptoms of significant end-organ dysfunction.
- **B.** Major risk factors for development of preeclampsia include past history of preeclampsia, pregestational diabetes, chronic hypertension, and autoimmune disease.
- **C.** The pathologic changes are present long before clinical manifestations.
- **D.** Endothelial dysfunction and disturbed angiogenic balance are one of the key features of the disease.
- **E.** Preeclampsia serum levels of VEGF, PLGF, PP13, and inhibin A are decreased, and sFlt-1 and sEng are increased.

8. Conclusions

Many studies demonstrate the importance of optimal management of blood pressure in pregnancy hypertension. The use of angiogenic biomarkers gives us promising results for the prediction and diagnosis of preeclampsia, but there is still a lack of specific and reliable biomarkers to predict preeclampsia, particularly in the first trimester of pregnancy. New methods to isolate and characterize markers outside the protein field (lipids, nucleic acids, etc.) from serum/plasma/urine/saliva are useful.

Author details

Osredkar Joško[1,2]* and Kumer Kristina[1]

1 University Medical Centre Ljubljana, Clinical Institute of Clinical Chemistry and Biochemistry, Ljubljana, Slovenia

2 Faculty of Pharmacy, University of Ljubljana, Ljubljana, Slovenia

*Address all correspondence to: josko.osredkar@kclj.si

References

[1] ACOG. American College of Obstetricians and Gynecologists, issuing body. II. Title. [DNLM: 1. Hypertension, Pregnancy-Induced—Practice Guideline. 2013, WQ 244]; 2014

[2] Whelton PK, Carey RM, Aronow WS, Casey DE Jr, Collins KJ, Dennison Himmelfarb C, et al. 2017 ACC/AHA/AAPA/ABC/ACPM/AGS/APhA/ASH/ASPC/NMA/PCNA Guideline for the prevention, detection, evaluation, and management of high blood pressure in adults: Executive summary: A report of the American College of Cardiology/American Heart Association Task Force on Clinical Practice Guidelines. Hypertension. 2018;**71**:1269-1324

[3] Ahmad AS, Samuelsen SO. Hypertensive disorders in pregnancy and fetal death at different gestational lengths: A population study of 2121371 pregnancies. BJOG. 2012;**119**:1521-1528

[4] Lindheimer MD, Taler SJ, Cunningham FG. Hypertension in pregnancy. Journal of the American Society of Hypertension. 2010;**4**:68-78

[5] Brown MA, Lindheimer MD, de Swiet M, Van Assche A, Moutquin JM. The classification and diagnosis of the hypertensive disorders of pregnancy: Statement from the international society for the study of hypertension in pregnancy (ISSHP). Hypertension in Pregnancy. 2001;**20**:IX-XIV

[6] ACOG Practice Bulletin. Diagnosis and management of preeclampsia and eclampsia. Number 33, January 2002. Obstetrics and Gynecology. 2002;**99**:159-167

[7] Karumanchi SA. Angiogenic factors in preeclampsia: From diagnosis to therapy. Hypertension. 2016;**67**:1072-1079

[8] Roberts JM. Endothelial dysfunction in preeclampsia. Seminars in Reproductive Endocrinology. 1998;**16**:5-15

[9] Hausvater A, Giannone T, Sandoval YH, Doonan RJ, Antonopoulos CN, Matsoukis IL, et al. The association between preeclampsia and arterial stiffness. Journal of Hypertension. 2012;**30**:17-33

[10] Fisher SJ, McMaster M, Roberts M. The placenta in normal pregnancy and preeclampsia. In: Chesley's Hypertensive Disorders in Pregnancy. Amsterdam, the Netherlands: Academic Press, Elsevier; 2009

[11] Tranquilli AL, Dekker G, Magee L, Roberts J, Sibai BM, Steyn W, et al. The classification, diagnosis and management of the hypertensive disorders of pregnancy: A revised statement from the isshp. Pregnancy Hypertension. 2014;**4**:97-104

[12] Zhang W, Xu Q, Wu J, et al. Role of Src in vascular hyperpermeability induced by advanced glycation end products. Scientific Reports. 2015;**5**:14090. DOI: 10.1038/srep14090

[13] Weinstein L. Syndrome of hemolysis, elevated liver enzymes, and low platelet count: A severe consequence of hypertension in pregnancy. American Journal of Obstetrics and Gynecology. 1982;**142**(2):159-167

[14] Sibai BM. Diagnosis, controversies, and management of the syndrome of hemolysis, elevated liver enzymes, and low platelet count. Obstetrics and Gynecology. 2004;**103**(5(Pt. 1)):981-991

[15] Maynard SE, Karumanchi SA, Thadhani R. Hypertension and kidney disease in pregnancy. In: Brenner BM, editor. Brenner and Rector's The Kidney. 8th ed. Philadelphia, PA: WB Saunders; 2007

[16] NIfHaC Excellence. CG107 NICE Guideline: Hypertension in Pregnancy. 2012

[17] Levine RJ, Maynard SE, Qian C, Lim KH, England LJ, Yu KF, et al. Circulating angiogenic factors and the risk of preeclampsia. New England Journal of Medicine. 2004;**350**:672-683. DOI: 10.1056/NEJMoa031884

[18] Kar M. Role of biomarkers in early detection of preeclampsia. Journal of Clinical and Diagnostic Research. 2014;**8**:BE01-BE04. DOI: 10.7860/JCDR/2014/7969.4261

[19] Ahmad S, Ahmed A. Elevated placental soluble vascular endothelial growth factor receptor-1 inhibits angiogenesis in preeclampsia. Circulation Research. 2004;**95**:884-891. DOI: 10.1161/01.RES.0000147365.86159.f5

[20] Thadhani R, Hagmann H, Schaarschmidt W, Roth B, Cingoez T, Karunnanchi SA, et al. Removal of soluble fms-like tyrosine kinase-1 by dextran sulfate apheresis in preeclampsia. Journal of the American Society of Nephrology. 2016;**27**:903-913. DOI: 10.1681/ASN.2015020157

[21] Jim B, Karumanchi SA. Preeclampsia: Pathogenesis, prevention, and long-term complications. Seminars in Nephrology. 2017;**37**:386-397. DOI: 10.1016/j.semnephrol.2017.05.011

[22] Iwasaki H, Kawamoto A, Tjwa M, Horii M, Hayashi S, Oyamada A, et al. PlGF repairs myocardial ischemia through mechanisms of angiogenesis, cardioprotection and recruitment of myo-angiogenic competent marrow progenitors. PLoS One. 2011;**6**:e24872. DOI: 10.1371/journal.pone.0024872

[23] De Falco S. The discovery of placenta growth factor and its biological activity. Experimental & Molecular Medicine. 2012;**44**:1-9. DOI: 10.3858/emm.2012.44.1.025

[24] Taylor RN, Grimwood J, Taylor RS, McMaster MT, Fisher SJ, North RA. Longitudinal serum concentrations of placental growth factor: Evidence for abnormal placental angiogenesis in pathologic pregnancies. American Journal of Obstetrics and Gynecology. 2003;**188**:177-182. DOI: 10.1067/mob.2003.111

[25] George EM, Granger JP. Recent insights into the pathophysiology of preeclampsia. Expert Review of Obstetrics & Gynecology. 2010;**5**:557-566. DOI: 10.1586/eog.10.45

[26] Staff AC, Benton SJ, von Dadelszen P, Roberts JM, Taylor RN, Powers RW, et al. Redefining preeclampsia using placenta-derived biomarkers. Hypertension. 2013;**61**:932-942. DOI: 10.1161/HYPERTENSIONAHA.111.00250

[27] Zeisler H, Llurba E, Chantraine F, Vatish M, Staff AC, Sennström M, et al. Predictive value of the sFlt-1:PlGF ratio in women with suspected preeclampsia. The New England Journal of Medicine. 2016;**374**:13-22. DOI: 10.1056/NEJMoa1414838

[28] Gregory AL, Xu G, Sotov V, Letarte M. Review: The enigmatic role of endoglin in the placenta. Placenta. 2014;**35**:S93-S99. DOI: 10.1016/j.placenta.2013.10.020

[29] Venkatesha S, Toporsian M, Lam C, Hanai J, Mammoto T, Kim YM, et al. Soluble endoglin contributes to the pathogenesis of preeclampsia. Nature Medicine. 2006;**12**:642-649. DOI: 10.1038/nm1429

[30] Robinson CJ, Johnson DD. Soluble endoglin as a second trimester marker for preeclampsia. American Journal of Obstetrics and Gynecology. 2007;**197**:174.e1-174.e5. DOI: 10.1016/j.ajog.2007.03.058

[31] Stepan H, Herraiz I, Schlembach S, Verlohren S, Brennecke S, Chantraine F, et al. Implementation of the sFlt-1/PlGF ratio for prediction and diagnosis of pre-eclampsia in singleton pregnancy: Implications for clinical practice. Ultrasound in Obstetrics & Gynecology. 2015;**45**:241-246

[32] Engels T, Pape J, Schoofs K, Henrich W, Verlohren S. Automated measurement of sFlt1, PlGF and sFlt1/PlGF ratio in differential diagnosis of hypertensive pregnancy disorders. Hypertension in Pregnancy. 2013;**32**(4):459-473

[33] Levine RJ, Lam C, Qian C, Yu KF, Maynard SE, Sachs BP, et al. Soluble endoglin and other circulating antiangiogenic factors in preeclampsia. New England Journal of Medicine. 2006;**355**(10):992-1005

[34] Jank A, Schaarschmidt W, Stepan H. Effect of steroids on angiogenic factors in pregnant women with HELLP syndrome. Journal of Perinatal Medicine. 2011;**39**:611-613

[35] Sahay AS, Jadhav AT, Sundrani DP, Wagh GN, Mehendale SS, Chavan-Gautam P, et al. VEGF and VEGFR1 levels in different regions of the normal and preeclampsia placentae. Molecular and Cellular Biochemistry. 2018;**438**(1-2):141-152

[36] Kumer K, Premru-Sršen T, Fabjan-Vodušek V, Tul N, Fabjan T, Osredkar J. Peripheral arterial tonometry and angiogenic biomarkers in preeclampsia. Hypertension in Pregnancy. 2018;(4):1-17

[37] Dymara-Konopka W, Laskowska M, Blazewicz A. Angiogenic imbalance as a contributor of preeclampsia. Current Pharmaceutical Biotechnology. 2018;**25**. DOI: 10.2174/138920101966618092511 5559

[38] Paiwattananupant K, Phupong V. Serum inhibin A level in preeclampsia and normotensive pregnancy. Hypertension in Pregnancy. 2008;**27**(4):337-343

[39] Huppertz B, Sammar M, Chefetz I, Neumaier-Wagner P, Bartz C, Meiri H. Longitudinal determination of serum placental protein 13 during development of preeclampsia. Fetal Diagnosis and Therapy. 2008;**24**(3):230-236

[40] Ferguson KK, McElrath TF, Chen YH, Mukherjee B, Meeker JD. Longitudinal profiling of inflammatory cytokines and C-reactive protein during uncomplicated and preterm pregnancy. American Journal of Reproductive Immunology. 2014;**72**(3):326-336

[41] McElrath TF, Allred EN, Van Marter L, Fichorova RN, Leviton A, ELGAN Study Investigators. Perinatal systemic inflammatory responses of growth-restricted preterm newborns. Acta Paediatrica. 2013;**102**(10):e439-e442

[42] Visegrady B, Than NG, Kilar F, Sumegi B, Than GN, Bohn H. Homology modelling and molecular dynamics studies of human placental tissue protein 13 (galectin-13). Protein Engineering. 2001;**14**(11):875-880

[43] Than NG, Pick E, Bellyei S, et al. Functional analyses of placental protein 13/galectin-13. European Journal of Biochemistry. 2004;**271**(6):1065-1078

[44] Burger O, Pick E, Zwickel J, et al. Placental protein 13 (PP-13): Effects on cultured trophoblasts, and its detection in human body fluids in normal and pathological pregnancies. Placenta. 2004;**25**(7):608-622

[45] Giudice LC, Conover CA, Bale L, et al. Identification and regulation of the IGFBP-4 protease and its physiological inhibitor in human trophoblasts and endometrial stroma: Evidence for paracrine regulation of IGF-II bioavailability in the placental

bed during human implantation. The Journal of Clinical Endocrinology and Metabolism. 2002;**87**(5):2359-2366

[46] Hamilton GS, Lysiak JJ, Han VK, Lala PK. Autocrine-paracrine regulation of human trophoblast invasiveness by insulin-like growth factor (IGF)-II and IGF-binding protein (IGFBP)-1. Experimental Cell Research. 1998;**244**(1):147-156

[47] Spencer CA, Allen VM, Flowerdew G, Dooley K, Dodds L. Low levels of maternal serum PAPP-A in early pregnancy and the risk of adverse outcomes. Prenatal Diagnosis. 2008;**28**(11):1029-1036

[48] D'Anna R, Baviera G, Giordano D, et al. First trimester serum PAPP-A and NGAL in the prediction of late-onset pre-eclampsia. Prenatal Diagnosis. 2009;**29**(11):1066-1068

[49] Dennis Lo YM, Chiu RW. Prenatal diagnosis: Progress through plasma nucleic acids. Nature Reviews. Genetics. 2007;**8**(1):71-77

[50] Maddocks DG, Alberry MS, Attilakos G, et al. The SAFE project: Towards non-invasive prenatal diagnosis. Biochemical Society Transactions. 2009;**37**(Pt. 2):460-465

[51] Lo YM, Leung TN, Tein MS, et al. Quantitative abnormalities of fetal DNA in maternal serum in preeclampsia. Clinical Chemistry. 1999;**45**(2):184-188

[52] Zhong XY, Holzgreve W, Hahn S. The levels of circulatory cell free fetal DNA in maternal plasma are elevated prior to the onset of preeclampsia. Hypertension in Pregnancy. 2002;**21**(1):77-83

[53] Leung TN, Zhang J, Lau TK, Chan LY, Lo YM. Increased maternal plasma fetal DNA concentrations in women who eventually develop preeclampsia. Clinical Chemistry. 2001;**47**(1):137-139

[54] Farina A, Sekizawa A, Iwasaki M, Matsuoka R, Ichizuka K, Okai T. Total cell-free DNA (beta-globin gene) distribution in maternal plasma at the second trimester: A new prospective for preeclampsia screening. Prenatal Diagnosis. 2004;**24**(9):722-726

[55] Valino N, Giunta G, Gallo DM, Akolekar R, Nicolaides KH. Biophysical and biochemical markers at 30-34 weeks' gestation in the prediction of adverse perinatal outcome. Ultrasound in Obstetrics & Gynecology. 2016;**47**:194-202

[56] Valiño N, Giunta G, Gallo DM, Akolekar R, Nicolaides KH. Biophysical and biochemical markers at 35-37 weeks' gestation in the prediction of adverse perinatal outcome. Ultrasound in Obstetrics & Gynecology. 2016;**47**(2): 203-209

[57] Duncan JR, Tobiasz AM, Bursac Z, Rios-Doria EV, Schenone MH, Mari G. Uterine artery flow velocity waveforms before and after delivery in hypertensive disorders of pregnancy near term. Hypertension in Pregnancy. 2018;**37**(3):131-136

[58] Ferrazzi E, Stampalija T, Monasta L, Di Martino D, Vonck S, Gyselaers W. Maternal hemodynamics: A method to classify hypertensive disorders of pregnancy. American Journal of Obstetrics and Gynecology. 2018;**218**(1):124.e1-124.e11

[59] Espinoza J, Romero R, Nien JK, et al. Identification of patients at risk for early onset and/or severe preeclampsia with the use of uterine artery Doppler velocimetry and placental growth factor. American Journal of Obstetrics and Gynecology. 2007;**196**(4):326e1-326e13

[60] Stepan H, Unversucht A, Wessel N, Faber R. Predictive value of maternal angiogenic factors in second trimester pregnancies with abnormal

uterine perfusion. Hypertension. 2007;**49**(4):818-824

[61] Stepan H, Geipel A, Schwarz F, Kramer T, Wessel N, Faber R. Circulatory soluble endoglin and its predictive value for preeclampsia in second-trimester pregnancies with abnormal uterine perfusion. American Journal of Obstetrics and Gynecology. 2008;**198**(2):175e1-175e6

[62] Nicolaides KH, Bindra R, Turan OM, et al. A novel approach to first-trimester screening for early pre-eclampsia combining serum PP-13 and Doppler ultrasound. Ultrasound in Obstetrics & Gynecology. 2006;**27**(1):13-17

[63] Spencer K, Cowans NJ, Chefetz I, Tal J, Meiri H. First-trimester maternal serum PP-13, PAPP-A and second-trimester uterine artery Doppler pulsatility index as markers of pre-eclampsia. Ultrasound in Obstetrics & Gynecology. 2007;**29**(2):128-134

[64] Akolekar R, Syngelaki A, Beta J, Kocylowski R, Nicolaides KH. Maternal serum placental protein 13 at 11-13 weeks of gestation in preeclampsia. Prenatal Diagnosis. 2009;**29**(12):1103-1108

[65] Poon LC, Kametas NA, Maiz N, Akolekar R, Nicolaides KH. First-trimester prediction of hypertensive disorders in pregnancy. Hypertension. 2009;**53**(5):812-818

[66] O'Gorman N, Wright D, Syngelaki A, et al. Competing risks model in screening for preeclampsia by maternal factors and biomarkers at 11-13 weeks gestation. American Journal of Obstetrics and Gynecology. 2016;**214**(1):103e1-103e12

[67] Wu P, van den Berg C, Alfirevic Z, O'Brien S, Röthlisberger M, Baker PN, et al. Early pregnancy biomarkers in pre-eclampsia: A systematic review and meta-analysis. International Journal of Molecular Sciences. 2015;**16**(9): 23035-23056. DOI: 10.3390/ijms160923035

[68] Farina A, Sekizawa A, Purwosunu Y, et al. Quantitative distribution of a panel of circulating mRNA in preeclampsia versus controls. Prenatal Diagnosis. 2006;**26**(12):1115-1120

[69] Tsui NB, Lo YM. A microarray approach for systematic identification of placentalderived RNA markers in maternal plasma. Methods in Molecular Biology. 2008;**444**:275-289

[70] Okazaki S, Sekizawa A, Purwosunu Y, Farina A, Wibowo N, Okai T. Placenta-derived, cellular messenger RNA expression in the maternal blood of preeclamptic women. Obstetrics and Gynecology. 2007;**110**(5):1130-1136

[71] Blumenstein M, McMaster MT, Black MA, et al. A proteomic approach identifies early pregnancy biomarkers for preeclampsia: Novel linkages between a predisposition to preeclampsia and cardiovascular disease. Proteomics. 2009;**9**(11):2929-2945

[72] Buhimschi IA, Zhao G, Funai EF, et al. Proteomic profiling of urine identifies specific fragments of SERPINA1 and albumin as biomarkers of preeclampsia. American Journal of Obstetrics and Gynecology. 2008;**199**(5):551e1-551e16

[73] Buhimschi IA, Nayeri UA, Zhao G, et al. Protein misfolding, congophilia, oligomerization, and defective amyloid processing in preeclampsia. Science Translational Medicine. 2014;**6**(245):245ra92

[74] Dunn WB, Brown M, Worton SA, et al. Changes in the metabolic footprint of placental explant-conditioned culture medium identifies metabolic disturbances related to

hypoxia and pre-eclampsia. Placenta. 2009;**30**(11):974-980

[75] Kenny LC, Broadhurst D, Brown M, et al. Detection and identification of novel metabolomic biomarkers in preeclampsia. Reproductive Sciences. 2008;**15**(6):591-597

[76] Hamburg NM, Benjamin EJ. A more recent approach involves the assessment of endothelial dysfunction using an EndoPAT device. Assessment of endothelial function using digital pulse amplitude tonometry. Trends in Cardiovascular Medicine. 2009;**19**(1):6-11

Chapter 5

Autophagy in Preeclampsia

Priscila Rezeck Nunes, Leandro Gustavo de Oliveira, Mariana Romão Veiga and Maria Terezinha Serrão Peraçoli

Abstract

Autophagy may be involved in gestation complicated by preeclampsia (PE) due to the presence of placental lesions caused by hypoxia at fetomaternal interphase. Autophagy is a lysosomal degradation pathway, removing protein aggregates and organelles damaged and thereby maintaining cell integrity. In preeclampsia, deficient myometrial penetration by extravillous cytotrophoblast occurs during the first trimester of pregnancy, leading to placental insufficiency. Several placental functions, like nutrient and oxygen input to the fetus during pregnancy, might benefit or even rely on autophagy and related material recycling within the cell. Deficiency in autophagy mechanism has been correlated to inflammatory responses. Autophagy is regulated during placentation and appears to be a possible factor in the development of preeclampsia. In this chapter, we intend to discuss evidence on autophagy pathway in pregnancy and the crosstalk between autophagy and inflammation in preeclampsia.

Keywords: preeclampsia, autophagy, inflammasome, placenta, inflammation

1. Introduction

Autophagy is an intracellular degradation system conserved among eukaryotes [1] characterized as a natural defense mechanism capable to reduce damages related to inflammatory responses and infectious, neoplasia and degenerative diseases. Defects in this process are directly linked to several diseases [2, 3]. The main role of autophagy is to maintain cellular homeostasis by recycling intracellular materials. Cells under starvation or with organelle damage trigger the autophagy mechanism in order to clean their cytoplasm and restore a source of energy [4–6].There are three types of autophagy: microautopahgy, chaperone-mediated autophagy, and macroautophagy [7]. The most characteristic process of autophagy is the macroautophagy. This process is characterized by the creation of a double membrane compartment in the cytoplasm called phagophore. This structure develops into an autophagosome, a double lipid bilayer membrane-bound structure. The autophagosome merges with lysosomes leading to the autolysosome formation. Continuing the process of autophagy, the autolysosome is finally degenerated, releasing in the cytosol a number of monomers that can be reused by the cell as important sources of energy (**Figure 1**) [8, 9].

The beginning of the autophagy process is dependent on the inhibition of the mammalian target of rapamycin (mTOR) and then autophagy proteins become crucial to the completion of the cascade generated [5, 10]. In this manner, cells under sufficient nutrition or without structural damages maintain a state of activation of mTOR, keeping blocked the mechanism of autophagy. After being triggered, mTOR provides a catalytic subunit by two distinct multiprotein complexes,

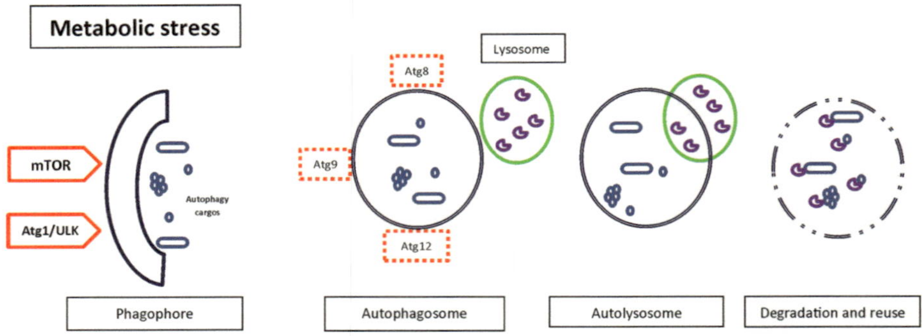

Figure 1.
Autolysosome formation. The process starts with a development of a double membrane named phagophore. This structure develops into an autophagosome, merging with lysosomes to form the autolysosome. During the process of autophagy, the autolysosome is degraded, releasing monomers into the cytosol, which can be reused by the cell as a source of energy. Source: own authorship.

mTORC1 (mechanistic target of rapamycin complex 1), and mTORC2 (mechanistic target of rapamycin complex 2). Some proteins are common for both complexes (GβL and Deptor), but others reflect specific functions for each of them, as raptor for mTORC1 and rictor for mTORC2 [11]. Regarding functions, mTORC1 coordinates the synthesis of lipids and proteins to promote cell growth, while mTORC2 acts in the cytoskeletal actin control [12]. Therefore, mTORC1 complex finally establishes the autophagy process via ULK1 (mammalian ortholog of yeast autophagy-related gene 1) kinase activity. The process of autophagosome formation involves about 38 Atgs (autophagy-related genes), and the initial process of autophagy in mammals is controlled by Atg1/ULK complex, which consists in ULK1/2 (UNC-51-like kinase 1), mAtg13, FIP200 (interaction protein of 200KD, homolog of the yeast Atg17), and Atg101. During nutrient rich conditions or in the presence of cell integrity, mTORC1 phosphorylates and inhibits ULK1/2 and mAtg13, deregulating the contact between ULK and AMPK (AMP-activated protein kinase), a kinase with activation effect on ULK1. But under altered conditions, mTORC1 is inhibited, and the activation of ULK1/2 leads to phosphorylation and activation of mAtg13 and FIP200 [13].

Atg plays crucial roles as ubiquitin-like protein conjugation system that mediates protein lipidation and participation in autophagy-specific protein kinase complexes [14, 15] for accomplishment of autophagy. Atg1 and Atg12-Atg5 complexes are essential for the autophagic machinery. Another important gene is Atg8 (a yeast autophagy-related gene ortholog of LC3), a membrane marker during the formation of autophagosome. Atg9 transmembrane protein and regulators of its trafficking (Atg2 and Atg18) participate in the expansion of phagophore after the formation of the Atg1 complex. There are two systems, Atg12 (Atg5, Atg7, Atg10, Atg12, and Atg16) and Atg8 (Atg3, Atg4, Atg7, and Atg8), which are responsible for expansion of the vesicle [1, 16].

The establishment of the autophagy is also dependent of two proteins: beclin-1 protein and LC3 (light chain protein 3) [17, 18]. Beclin-1 (homolog of yeast Apg6/Vps30) promotes the recruitment of membranes to form the autophagosome, nucleation of the autophagic vesicle, and recruitment of proteins from the cytosol [19]. Three isoforms of LC3 have been described: LC3A, LC3B, and LC3C. After synthesis and activation (LC3-I to LC3-II), LC3-II for incorporating cytosolic denatured proteins and damaged organelles into the autophagosome [20, 21]. The relative amounts of LC3-II reflect autophagic activity [22]. Considering the autophagy pathway, LC3-II has been proposed to be used to measure autophagy activity.

Defective autophagy caused by mutations or genetic alterations can lead to various clinical syndromes [23], such as static encephalopathy of childhood with neurodegeneration in adulthood (SENDA), Vici syndrome, hereditary spastic paraparesis, Parkinson's disease, lysosomal storage disorders, cancer, and Crohn's disease.

As a lysosomal degradation pathway, removing protein aggregates and organelles damaged, maintaining cell integrity, autophagy may be impaired in pregnant women with preeclampsia (PE) due to the presence of placental lesions caused by hypoxia/ischemia [24]. In preeclampsia, there is deficient myometrial penetration by extravillous cytotrophoblast during the first trimester of pregnancy, leading to placental insufficiency [25]. On the other hand, it has been reported that proteins related to autophagy, LC3-II, and beclin-1 are present in trophoblastic villi during normal pregnancy, and high levels of LC3-II are present in the placenta of pregnant women with severe preeclampsia [26]. The induction of hypoxia on choriocarcinoma cell line JEG-3 with the purpose of exploring the mechanism of regulatory proteins involved in autophagy showed a slight increase in the expression of LC3-II, with a reduction in beclin-1. Treatment of these cells with TNF-α induced a significant increase in the expression of LC3-II without modifying the expression of beclin-1. The results suggest that the increased autophagic activity mediated by LC3-II may be involved in the pathophysiology of preeclampsia [26].

Studies with autophagy in the placenta are scarce, and most of the work done employs cell lines or cultures of trophoblast cells in vitro to evaluate autophagy induced by nutrient deprivation and oxygen [27].

The systemic inflammatory response exacerbated in preeclampsia seems to be related to the release of substances capable of inducing inflammation as membrane fragments of syncytiotrophoblast, fetal DNA, soluble microparticles derived from leukocytes, and inflammatory cytokines in plasma of pregnant women, causing activation of cells of innate immunity [28–30]. Other cellular components present in plasma, such as protein derivatives, polysaccharides, and lipids, as well as extracellular matrix products are named "damage-associated molecular patterns" (DAMPS) and are considered important modulators of the inflammatory response. DAMPs are represented by molecules like uric acid, reactive oxygen intermediates, heat shock proteins (Hsp) [31], proteins released from dead cells, as the high mobility group box 1—HMGB1 [32], and products released from the extracellular matrix, such as fibronectin and hyaluronan [33, 34]. Both protein hsp70 [35, 36] and hyaluronan [37, 38] are elevated in plasma of pregnant women with preeclampsia and may be associated with systemic inflammation and oxidative stress. However, the role of these factors in the pathophysiology of preeclampsia is not well understood. A major cause of preeclampsia is the accumulation of reactive oxygen species (ROS), resulting in impaired antioxidant protection and activation of autophagy. According to research in trophoblasts, expression of LC3 and beclin-1 and the formation of autophagosomes are higher than in normal placentas, suggesting that autophagy is regulated during placentation and appears to be a possible factor in the development of preeclampsia [39].

2. Autophagy and placenta

The placental development requires multiples roles of autophagy. Experimental studies suggest that autophagy plays important functions in survival of neonates during nutritional deficiency at the early stage of birth [40]. Moreover, it was seen that the growth and remodeling of cervical fascia progress by autophagy regulation. Meanwhile, it has not been reported that autophagy affects differentiation of trophoblasts in pregnant women by LC3-II and beclin-1, markers which are analyzed and compared between term placentas, and in their first trimester of gestation [39]. Autophagy is essential for placental development and for maintaining pregnancy, and the disruption of autophagy in extravillous trophoblast (EVT) contributes to hypoplastic placentation. Placentas of patients with preeclampsia present high levels of autophagy, with lower LC3 activation, and higher apoptosis than normal pregnancies. When induced by external factors such as hypoxia, autophagy directly affects trophoblast infiltration during normal placental development [41].

The study of autophagy markers in preeclampsia demonstrated that there are different patterns during normal pregnancy and preeclampsia, in part, because of the environmental factors, like hypoxia. Cells exposed to hypoxic conditions demonstrated higher levels of LC3, beclin-1, and the autophagosome formation when compared to normal placentas. Saito and Nakashima [24] reported that poor placentation is induced by decreased infiltration of trophoblasts due to abnormal processing for autophagy, which is activated by soluble endoglin (sENG). Inactivation of autophagy represses trophoblast infiltration and vascular remodeling due to excessive hypoxia, causing poor placentation, as observed in preeclampsia [26]. Hung and collaborators showed that autophagy decreased with advancing of gestational age in placentas of normotensive women, through analyses of changes in LC3-II and p62 according to gestational weeks [42].

The determination of p62 levels also has a few reports and in addition with the analysis of LC3-II [2, 14, 43] may be important to determine autophagic status in the villous tissue.

This important finding has been the basis of several investigations on oxidative stress, an alteration identified in placental related disorders, and whether this oxidative stress is able to induce autophagy activation on placental explants. We developed an in vitro study with the objective of evaluating the effect of oxidative stress induced by hydrogen peroxide (H_2O_2) on the occurrence of autophagy activation in placental explants of pregnant women at term (39–40 weeks), without clinical or obstetric disorders identified and undergone to elective cesarean section. In the methodology, we intended to reproduce experimentally the pathophysiology of obstetric complications related to placental dysfunction caused by uterine circulatory alterations. These alterations are responsible for the establishment of the hypoxia-reoxygenation phenomenon also called as ischemia-reperfusion injury and consequent production of (ROS).

The results showed the higher gene expression of LC3-II, beclin-1, and p62 detected in cultures exposed to different concentrations of H_2O_2 and demonstrated that the oxidative stress generated was able to induce autophagy in placental explants (**Figure 2**). Material and methods of this experiment are shown as supplementary material to this chapter.

Gene expression of LC3-II (**Figure 2A**) was increased in tissues exposed to the concentration of 1000 μM of H_2O_2 compared to the non-exposed cultures, which means that autophagy was more activated in this concentration, in response to the oxidative effect. Gene expression of beclin-1 and p62 (**Figure 2B** and **C**) increased in front of increasing concentrations of H_2O_2 with the maximum value in 1000 μM of H_2O_2, showing statistical difference ($p < 0.05$) when compared to controls.

In the present study, the higher gene expression of LC3-II, beclin-1, and p62 detected in cultures exposed to H_2O_2 demonstrated that the oxidative stress generated was able to induce autophagy in placental explants.

The high expressions of mRNA for LC3-II and TNF-α (**Figure 3A** and **B**) demonstrated in our study corroborate with other reports, showing that placental

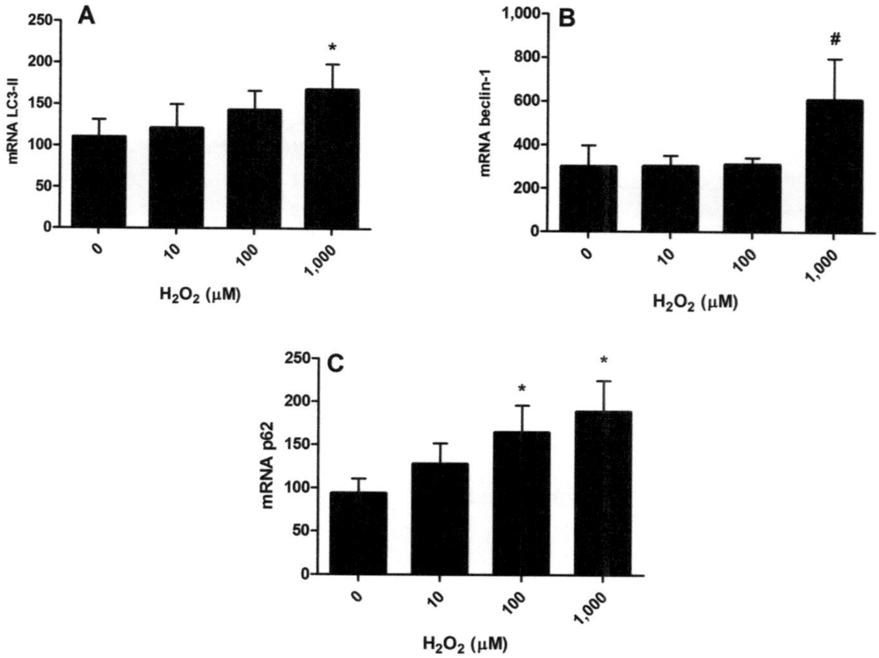

Figure 2.
*Activation of autophagy in cultures exposed to different concentrations of hydrogen peroxide. mRNA expression of LC3-II (A), beclin-1 (B), and p62 (C) in placental explants. Results expressed as mean ± SD. * ($p < 0.05$) vs. 0; # ($p < 0.05$) vs. 0, 10, 100 μM (ANOVA). Source: own authorship.*

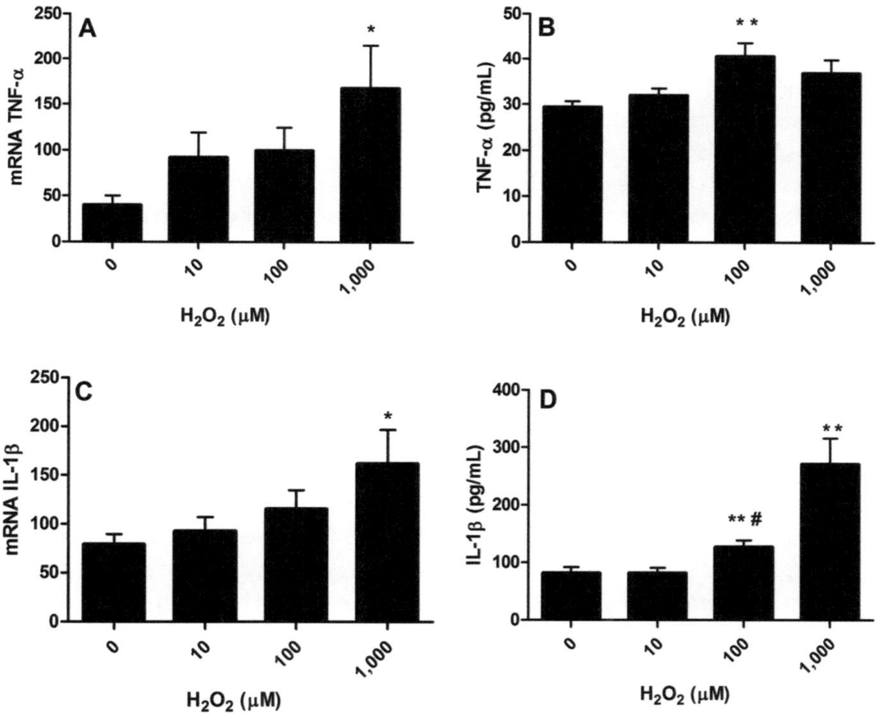

Figure 3.
*Pro-inflammatory cytokine profile in cultures exposed to different concentrations of hydrogen peroxide. Gene and protein expression of pro-inflammatory cytokines TNF-α(A/B) and IL-1β (C/D) in placental explants. Results expressed as mean ± SD. * ($p < 0.05$) vs. 0 (ANOVA). Source: own authorship.*

hypoxic environment and the presence of TNF-α caused a positive regulation in the autophagy-related protein LC3-II in a trophoblastic cell line [26].

Gene expressions of TNF-α and IL-1β were higher in explants cultured with 1000 μM of H_2O_2 with significant difference ($p < 0.05$) to culture without H_2O_2 (**Figure 3A** and **C**). The protein expressions of these cytokines (**Figure 3B** and **D**) were higher in the supernatants from concentrations of 100 to 1000 μM of H_2O_2, with difference ($p < 0.05$) to non-exposed and cultures with 10 μM of H_2O_2. The protein expression of IL-1 β was higher in 1000 μM of H_2O_2 ($p < 0.05$) than in the culture of 100 μM of H_2O_2 (**Figure 3D**).

The similar patterns of p62, beclin-1, and LC3-II gene expressions suggest the production of mRNA for the p62 protein transcription, which will be degraded during autophagy activation. This protein plays a significant role on the regulation of oxidative stress, degenerative diseases, and carcinogenesis [44].

3. Autophagy and inflammasomes

Inflammasome is a molecular platform composed of nucleotide-binding oligomerization domain (NOD)-like receptor (NLR) proteins. It is required for the activation of caspase-1 and subsequent maturation of the pro-inflammatory cytokines interleukin-1β and IL-18 [45]. NLRs respond to different endogenous or exogenous stimuli and activate caspase-1. During inflammation, these pro-inflammatory molecules are maturated in inflammasomes, which are in part regulated by the autophagy mechanism.

Actually, autophagy can control endogenous inflammasome activators, such as pro-IL-1β, which regulates the secretion of IL-1β and IL-18, thereby preventing an exaggerated inflammation [9, 45, 46].The activation of the inflammasome NLRP3 occurs via two signals: the first signal is provided by NF-kB activators and is a prerequisite for inflammasome activation via NLRP3 expression in macrophages [47]; the second signal activates NLRP3 inflammasome directly and involves host-derived adenosine triphosphate (ATP), uric acid crystals, bacterial toxins, or particulate matter (**Figure 4**) [48].

Some studies have demonstrated a mutual relationship between autophagy and inflammasomes. Autophagy negatively regulates inflammasome activation. Autophagy induction is dependent on the presence of specific inflammasome sensors, inflammasomes are ultimately degraded by autophagosomes via the selective autophagic receptor p62, and autophagy plays a role in the biogenesis and secretion of the pro-inflammatory cytokine IL-1β [45, 9, 49].

The role of autophagy in inflammasome regulation may depend on the context of danger signal. In the absence of a danger signal, autophagy can act removing IL-1β and inflammasome components while maintaining cellular homeostasis. In the presence of a danger signal, autophagy may act initially as a secretory pattern to diffuse inflammation while preventing cell death and pyroptosis. Recent studies showed that macrophages may activate autophagy in response to inflammasome activation, as a way to delay the onset of pyroptosis. According to the authors, the inhibition of autophagy resulted in increased activation of pyroptosis and the impact of these types of cell death regulation by autophagy need to be more studied on inflammatory process [50]. When genes of autophagy regulator Atg 16L1 or Atg7 are deleted or a chemical inhibitor of autophagy is applied, LPS-dependent inflammasome activation occurs suggesting that autophagy controls inflammasome activation and can limit production of cytokines IL-1β and IL-18 [51]. Induced autophagy to inhibit the inflammasome and excessive inflammation or marking directly specific NLRs (NOD-like

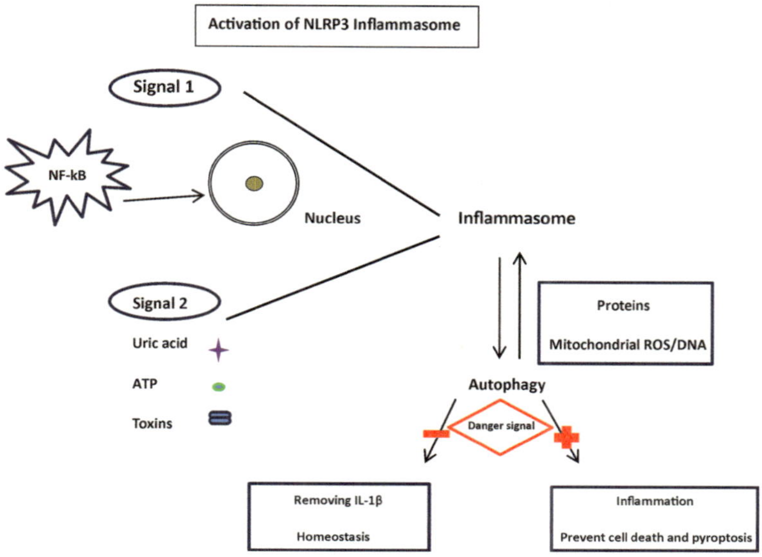

Figure 4.
Activation of NLRP3 inflammasome. This process requires two signals: the first is dependent of NF-kB activators and the second demands ATP, uric acid crystals, bacterial toxins or particulate matter to activate NLRP3 inflammasome. Source: own authorship.

receptors) to reduce its activity may be a promising strategy to reverse inflammatory process [52].

In the present study, the oxidative stress induced by H_2O_2 on placental explants contributed to the inflammatory profile generated by activating the NLRP3 inflammasome, caspase-1 and inducing the release of IL-1β (**Figure 3C** and **D**).

In a previous study published by our research group, we observed that some markers of oxidative stress, such as superoxide dismutase (SOD) and catalase are altered at high concentrations of hydrogen peroxide confirming that H_2O_2 induces oxidative stress on placental explants and demonstrated that this stress involves inflammasome activation [53].

We demonstrated that gene expressions of NLRP3 and caspase-1 have similar patterns, with greater expression in cultures exposed to the concentration of 1000 μM of H_2O_2, which means that this concentration was able to activate the NLRP3 inflammasome (**Figure 5**). The activation of this complex may occur as a

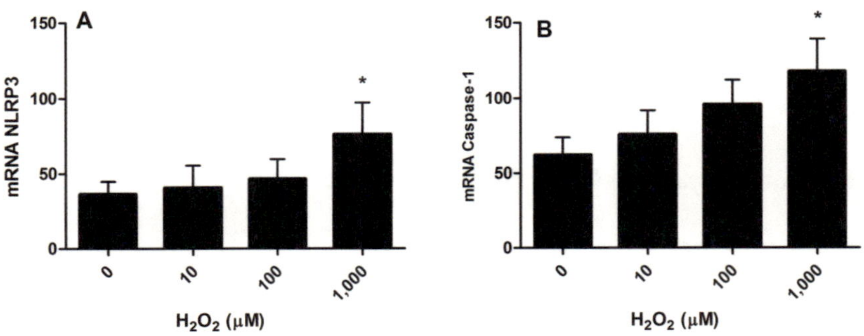

Figure 5.
*Inflammasome activation in placental explants in cultures exposed to different concentrations of hydrogen peroxide. mRNA expression of NLRP3 (A) and caspase-1 (B) in explants of placental explants. Results expressed as mean ± SD. * (p < 0.05) vs. 0, 10 μM (ANOVA). Source: own authorship.*

consequence of a common form of cellular stress initiated by different stimuli, such as the release of ROS [54, 55].

The relationship between occurrence of inflammasome and autophagy activation may be explained by the elevation in gene expression of p62 under conditions of oxidative stress. Inflammasome can be degraded by autophagosomes through this protein [56].

4. Conclusion

Taken together, the results of the present study confirm that H_2O_2 induces oxidative stress in placental explants, demonstrated by activation of NLRP3 inflammasome, which in turn induce the autophagy activation in order to control the inflammatory state. Activation of inflammasome and autophagy are essential elements of the innate immune system, and disorders in these processes have been implicated in various inflammatory and infectious diseases [57]. Oxidative stress may also contribute to placental tissue senescence and to the pathophysiology of some placental-related disorders of pregnancy, such as preeclampsia and fetal growth restriction [56]. Thus, initiatives to reduce stress on trophoblastic tissue should be considered for future researches.

Many studies have observed the effects of supplementation to prevent the effects of oxidative stress and autophagy in preeclampsia, such as the use of antioxidants, vitamins C and E, calcium, resveratrol and some natural products [58–61].

The use of natural products and hormones such as Vitamin D may be a new model to reduce inflammation by regulating autophagy, since there is a direct correlation between vitamin D levels and cell survival in pathologies associated with gestation. Vitamin D and its components such as vitamin D receptor (VDR) are molecules that are highly related to the autophagic process [62]. In this sense, the use of products with antioxidant and anti-inflammatory effects still need to be evaluated in order to reduce oxidative stress, induce autophagy, and decrease the activation of inflammasome in placental tissue.

Acknowledgements

Results showed in this chapter were supported by the Fundação de Amparo a Pesquisa do Estado de São Paulo, FAPESP (Grant No 2014/25611-5).

Conflict of interest

The authors declare that they have no conflict of interest.

Supplementary material

1. Material and methods

1.1 Study population and ethics statement

This study consisted of 15 healthy pregnant women with normal evolution of the pregnancy, with no personal history of hypertensive disorders in pregnancy. These pregnant women were admitted to the Obstetrics Unit of Botucatu Medical School,

Sao Paulo State University, Botucatu, SP, Brazil between November 2015 and May 2016. Gestational age was calculated from the last menstrual period and confirmed by ultrasound dating. Exclusion criteria included chronic hypertension, multiple gestation, prior preeclampsia, illicit drug use, and preexisting medical conditions such as diabetes, cancer, acute infectious disease, cardiovascular, autoimmune, renal and hepatic diseases. The study was approved by the Ethics Committee of the Botucatu Medical School, and written informed consent was obtained from all women involved in the study (CAAE Protocol number: 37160614500005411).

1.2 Collection of placental tissue

All placentas from normotensive pregnant women were delivered by cesarean section, without labor and were examined macroscopically and processed within 10 min of delivery. Fragments of approximately 5 × 5 cm were immediately removed from the central region of the placenta, constituting samples of the villous cytotrophoblast and the syncytiotrophoblast region in contact with the maternal side (basal plate). After collection, the trophoblastic tissue was washed in buffered saline (PBS) and separated from the decidual layer that is normally adhered to the basal plate. The terminal portions of the villi were evidenced in PBS (the villi were seen floating freely in the liquid) and dissected in small sections to constitute explants.

1.3 Culture of placental explants with hydrogen peroxide

The amount of villi used was 11 mg of placental tissue that was cultured in each well of 24-well plates (SPL Life Sciences, Korea) for 24 h for stabilization [63]. Cultures were performed in vitro in the absence of hydrogen peroxide or in the presence of 10, 100, and 1,000 μM of H_2O_2 for 4 h and 24 h in RPMI 1640 culture medium supplemented with 2 mM L-glutamine (Sigma-Aldrich, St Louis, MO, USA), 40 mg/ml antibiotic/antimycotic (Sigma-Aldrich), and 10% fetal bovine serum (Gibco BRL Life Technologies, The Netherlands) inactivated (complete RPMI medium).

After the culture periods, the explants were removed and submitted to RNA extraction for further analysis of the expression of genes related to inflammation (cytokines), autophagy, and inflammasome. Culture supernatants were obtained, centrifuged at 2,000 g for 10 min and stored at −80°C for determination of cytokines.

1.4 Cell viability assay

The cell viability assay was conducted through the activity of the enzyme lactate dehydrogenase (LDH) in supernatants of placental explant after 24, 48, 72, and 96 h of culture and was determined by commercial kit (Sigma-Aldrich) according to the manufacturer's instructions.

1.5 Evaluation of the expression of transcripts related to inflammation

The placental explants were evaluated for the expression of the genes encoding IL-1β, TNF-α, LC3-II, beclin-1, and p62 proteins at the transcriptional level. In addition, the gene expression of the inflammasome was evaluated through the NLRP3 and caspase-1 genes. Total RNA was extracted from the placentas using the Total RNA Purification Kit (Norgen Biotek Corp., Thorold, Canada) according to the manufacturer's protocol, and the Reverse Transcription-coupled polymerase chain reaction (RT-qPCR) was performed as described previously [64]. Briefly, isolated RNA was DNAse I Amp Grade (Invitrogen) treated. Subsequently, the synthesis of complementary DNA (cDNA) was conducted using ImProm-IITM Reverse Transcription System,

Gene	Sequence (5′-3′)	Name	GeneBank
Caspase-1	Forward primer: (1065) AGACATCCCACAATGGGCTC(1084) Reverse primer: (1172) TGAAAATCGAACCTTGCGGAAA(1151)	CASP1	NM_033292.3
NLRP3	Forward primer: (2826) GAGGAAAAGGAAGGCCGACA(2845) Reverse primer: (2917) TGGCTGTTCACCAATCCATGA(2897)	NLRP3	NM_004895.4
IL-1β	Forward primer: (544) GAGCAACAAGTGGTGTTCTCC(564) Reverse primer: (653) AACACGCAGGACAGGTACAG(634)	IL1B	NM_000576.2
TNF-α	Forward primer: (325) GCTGCACTTTGGAGTGATCG(344) Reverse primer: (462) GGGTTTGCTACAACATGGGC(443)	TNF	NM_000594.3
p62	Forward primer: (159) CGCTTCAGCTTCTGCTGC(176) Reverse primer: (308) GTCCTCATCGCGGTAGTGC(290)	SQSTM1	NM_003900.4
Beclin-1	Forward primer: (101) GTAGACCGGACTTGGGTGAC(120) Reverse primer: (198) CATGGTGCTGTTGTTGGACG(179)	BECN1	NM_003766.3
LC3-II	Forward primer: (517) CCAGGAAACCTTCGGCTTCT(536) Reverse primer: (632) CGGTAGAGGCAGCTCAGTTC(613)	MP1LC3A	NM_032514.3
GAPDH	Forward primer: (684) CGTGGAAGGACTCATGACCA(703) Reverse primer: (801) GGCAGGGATGATGTTCTGGA(782)	GAPDH	NM_002046.4

Table 1.
Primers for inflammasome and autophagy proteins, cytokines, and GAPDH. Source: Gen Bank (https://www.ncbi.nlm.nih.gov/genbank).

according to manufacturer's protocol. The RT-qPCR was made using RT GoTaq-qPCR Master Mix (Promega, Madison, WI, USA), and the primer sequences used in this study are listed in **Table 1**. Each reaction was set in duplicate and the conditions for the RT-qPCR were as follows: initial denaturation at 96°C for 2 min and then 40 cycles at 95°C for 15 s and 60°C for 60 s, followed by a melting curve. Expression values of the analyzed transcripts were normalized to that of the enzyme-encoding glyceraldehyde-3-phosphate dehydrogenase gene (GAPDH).

The calculation of the differential expression of selected genes was carried out by the data processing method compared with a standard curve [65]. To analyze relative gene expression, we standardized the RNA expression levels in all samples to that of a single RNA sample, which was set to a value of 100.

1.6 Cytokine determination

Cytokine concentrations in culture supernatants of placental explants were determined by enzyme-linked immunosorbent assay (ELISA), using Quantikine

ELISA kits (R&D Systems) for TNF-α and IL-1β according to the manufacturer's instructions. Assay sensitivity limits were 1.6 pg./mL for TNF-α and 3.9 pg./mL for IL-1β.

1.7 Statistical Analysis

All of the data were analyzed using one-way ANOVA, followed by post-hoc Tukey test using the statistical program PRISM (Graph Prism for Windows, version 6.01, GraphPad, EUA) to compare the difference among the groups. A p value less than 0.05 was considered to be statistically significant.

Key points

1. Autophagy is an intracellular degradation system characterized as a natural defense mechanism capable to reduce damages related to inflammatory responses.

2. The main role of autophagy is to maintain cellular homeostasis by recycling intracellular materials.

3. Activation of inflammasome and autophagy are essential elements of the innate immune system, and disorders in these processes have been implicated in various inflammatory and infectious diseases.

4. Oxidative stress may also contribute to placental tissue senescence and to the pathophysiology of some placental-related disorders of pregnancy, such as preeclampsia and fetal growth restriction.

5. The use of products with antioxidant and anti-inflammatory effects still need to be evaluated in order to reduce oxidative stress, induce autophagy, and decrease the activation of inflammasome in placental tissue.

Author details

Priscila Rezeck Nunes*, Leandro Gustavo de Oliveira, Mariana Romão Veiga and Maria Terezinha Serrão Peraçoli
Sao Paulo State University—UNESP, Botucatu, Brazil

*Address all correspondence to: priscilarezeck@gmail.com

References

[1] Mizushima N, Yoshimori T, Ohsumi Y. The role of Atg proteins in autophagosome formation. Annual Review of Cell and Developmental Biology. 2011;**27**:107-132. DOI: 10.1146/annurev-cellbio-092910-154005

[2] Jiang P, Mizushima N. LC3- and p62-based biochemical methods for the analysis of autophagy progression in mammalian cells. Methods. 2014;**75**:18-22. DOI: 10.1016/j.ymeth.2014.11.021

[3] Mizushima N, Komatsu M. Autophagy: Renovation of cells and tissues. Cell. 2011;**147**:728-741. DOI: 10.1016/j.cell.2011.10.026

[4] Mizushima N, Levine B, Cuervo AM, Klionsky DJ. Autophagy fights disease through cellular self-digestion. Nature. 2008;**451**:1069-1075. DOI: 10.1038/nature06639

[5] Jo EK, Shin DM, Choi AMK. Autophagy: Cellular defense to excessive inflammation. Microbes and Infection. 2012;**14**:119-125. DOI: 10.1016/j.micinf.2011.08.014

[6] Mizushima N, Klionsky DJ. Protein turnover via autophagy: implications for metabolism. Annual Review of Nutrition. 2007;**27**:19-40. DOI: 10.1146/annurev.nutr.27.061406.093749

[7] Taylor P, Yue Y, Li J, Zhang S, Lin X, Chu J, et al. YY1-MIR372-SQSTM1 regulatory axis in autophagy. Autophagy. 2014;**10**:37-41. DOI: 10.4161/auto.29486.

[8] Mulakkal NC, Nagy P, Takats S, Tusco R, Juhász G, Nezis IP. Autophagy in drosophila: From historical studies to current knowledge. BioMed Research International. 2014;**2014**:273473

[9] Levine B, Mizushima N, Virgin HW. Autophagy in immunity and inflammation. Nature. 2011;**469**:323-335. DOI: 10.1038/nature09782

[10] Dragowska WH, Weppler SA, Qadir MA, Wong LY, Franssen Y, Baker JHE, et al. The combination of gefitinib and RAD001 inhibits growth of HER2 overexpressing breast cancer cells and tumors irrespective of trastuzumab sensitivity. BMC Cancer. 2011;**11**:420. DOI: 10.1186/1471-2407-11-420

[11] Guertin DA, Stevens DM, Thoreen CC, Burds AA, Kalaany NY, Moffat J, et al. Ablation in mice of the mTORC components raptor, rictor, or mLST8 reveals that mTORC2 is required for signaling to Akt-FOXO and PKC a, but not S6K1. Developmental Cell. 2006;**11**(6):859-871. DOI: 10.1016/j.devcel.2006.10.007

[12] Jacinto E, Loewith R, Schmidt A, Lin S, Rüegg MA, Hall A, et al. Mammalian TOR complex 2 controls the actin cytoskeleton and is rapamycin insensitive. Nature Cell Biology. 2004;**6**(11):1122-1128. DOI: 10.1038/ncb1183

[13] Jung CH, Seo M, Otto NM, Kim D, Hwa C, Seo M, et al. ULK1 inhibits the kinase activity of mTORC1 and cell proliferation. Autophagy. 2011;**7**(10):1212-1221. DOI: 10.4161/auto.7.10.16660

[14] Ichimura Y, Komatsu M. Selective degradation of p62 by autophagy. Seminars in Immunopathology. 2010;**32**:431-436. DOI: 10.1007/s00281-010-0220-1

[15] Kamada Y, Funakoshi T, Shintani T, Nagano K, Ohsumi M, Ohsumi Y. Tor-mediated induction of autophagy via an Apg1 protein kinase complex. The Journal of Cell Biology. 2000;**150**(6):1507-1513. DOI: 10.1083/jcb.150.6.1507

[16] Klionsky DJ, Schulman BA. Dynamic regulation of macroautophagy by distinctive ubiquitin-like proteins. Nature Structural & Molecular Biology. 2014;**21**:336-345. DOI: 10.1038/nsmb.2787

[17] Levine B, Yuan J. Autophagy in cell death: An innocent convict? The Journal of Clinical Investigation. 2005;**115**:2679-2688. DOI: 10.1172/JCI26390

[18] Shintani T, Klionsky DJ. Autophagy in health and disease: A double-edged sword. Science. 2004;**306**:990-995. DOI: 10.1126/science.1099993

[19] Ferraro E, Cecconi F. Autophagic and apoptotic response to stress signals in mammalian cells. Archives of Biochemistry and Biophysics. 2007;**462**:210-219. DOI: 10.1016/j.abb.2007.02.006

[20] Lamark T, Kirkin V, Dikic I, Johansen T. NBR1 and p62 as cargo receptors for selective autophagy of ubiquitinated targets. Cell Cycle. 2009;**8**:1986-1990. DOI: 10.4161/cc.8.13.8892

[21] Yue Z, Jin S, Yang C, Levine AJ, Heintz N. Beclin 1, an autophagy gene essential for early embryonic development, is a haploinsufficient tumor suppressor. Proceedings of the National Academy of Sciences of the United States of America. 2003;**100**:15077-15082. DOI: 10.1073/pnas.2436255100

[22] Yorimitsu T, Klionsky DJ. Eating the endoplasmic reticulum: Quality control by autophagy. Trends in Cell Biology. 2007;**17**:279-285. DOI: 10.1016/j.tcb.2007.04.005

[23] Jiang P, Mizushima N. Autophagy and human diseases. Cell Research. 2014;**24**(1):69-79. DOI: 10.1038/cr.2013.161

[24] Saito S, Nakashima A. Review: The role of autophagy in extravillous trophoblast function under hypoxia. Placenta. 2013;**34**:S79-S84. DOI: 10.1016/j.placenta.2012.11.026

[25] Huppertz B. Placental origins of preeclampsia: Challenging the current hypothesis. Hypertension. 2008;**51**(4):970-975. DOI: 10.1161/HYPERTENSIONAHA.107.107607

[26] Oh S-Y, Choi S-J, Kim KH, Cho EY, Kim J-H, Roh C-R. Autophagy-related proteins, LC3 and Beclin-1, in placentas from pregnancies complicated by preeclampsia. Reproductive Sciences. 2008;**15**:912-920. DOI: 10.1177/1933719108319159

[27] Curtis S, Jones CJP, Garrod A, Hulme CH, Heazell AEP. Identification of autophagic vacuoles and regulators of autophagy in villous trophoblast from normal term pregnancies and in fetal growth restriction. Journal of Maternal-Fetal and Neonatal Medicine. 2012;**26**:1-8. DOI: 10.3109/14767058.2012.733764

[28] Redman CWG, Sargent IL. Pre-eclampsia, the placenta and the maternal systemic inflammatory response—A review. Placenta. 2003;**24**:21-27. DOI: 10.1053/plac.2002.0930

[29] Borzychowski AM, Sargent IL, Redman CWG. Inflammation and pre-eclampsia. Seminars in Fetal & Neonatal Medicine. 2006;**11**:309-316. DOI: 10.1016/j.siny.2006.04.001

[30] Lok CA, Jebbink J, Nieuwland R, Faas MM, Boer K, Sturk A, et al. Leukocyte activation and circulating leukocyte-derived microparticles in preeclampsia. American Journal of Reproductive Immunology. 2009;**61**:346-359. DOI: 10.1111/j.1600-0897.2009.00701.x

[31] Asea A, Rehli M, Kabingu E, Boch JA, Baré O, Auron PE, et al. Novel signal transduction pathway utilized

by extracellular HSP70. Role of toll-like receptor (TLR) 2 and TLR4, The Journal of Biological Chemistry 277 (2002) 15028-15034. doi:10.1074/jbc.M200497200

[32] Park JS, Svetkauskaite D, He Q, Kim J-Y, Strassheim D, Ishizaka A, et al. Involvement of toll-like receptors 2 and 4 in cellular activation by high mobility group box 1 protein. The Journal of Biological Chemistry. 2004;**279**:7370-7377. DOI: 10.1074/jbc.M306793200

[33] Okamura Y, Watari M, Jerud ES, Young DW, Ishizaka ST, Rose J, et al. The extra domain a of fibronectin activates toll-like receptor 4. The Journal of Biological Chemistry. 2001;**276**:10229-10233. DOI: 10.1074/jbc.M100099200

[34] Campo GM, Avenoso A, Campo S, D'Ascola A, Nastasi G, Calatroni A. Small hyaluronan oligosaccharides induce inflammation by engaging both toll-like-4 and CD44 receptors in human chondrocytes. Biochemical Pharmacology. 2010;**80**:480-490. DOI: 10.1016/j.bcp.2010.04.024

[35] Molvarec A, Rigó J, Lázár L, Balogh K, Makó V, Cervenak L, et al. Increased serum heat-shock protein 70 levels reflect systemic inflammation, oxidative stress and hepatocellular injury in preeclampsia. Cell Stress & Chaperones. 2009;**14**:151-159. DOI: 10.1007/s12192-008-0067-8

[36] Peraçoli JC, Bannwart-Castro CF, Romao M, Weel IC, Ribeiro VR, Borges VTM, et al. High levels of heat shock protein 70 are associated with pro-inflammatory cytokines and may differentiate early- from late-onset preeclampsia. Journal of Reproductive Immunology. 2013;**100**:129-134. DOI: 10.1016/j.jri.2013.08.003

[37] Romão M, Weel IC, Lifshitz SJ, Peraçoli MTS, Witkin SS. Elevated hyaluronan and extracellular matrix metalloproteinase inducer levels in women with preeclampsia. Archives of Gynecology and Obstetrics. 2014;**289**:575-579. DOI: 10.1007/s00404-013-3021-7

[38] Romão-Veiga M, Matias ML, Ribeiro VR, Nunes PR, Borges VTM, Peraçoli JC, et al. Induction of systemic inflammation by hyaluronan and hsp70 in women with pre-eclampsia. Cytokine. 2018;**105**:23-31. DOI: 10.1016/j.cyto.2018.02.007

[39] Gong J, Kim GJ. The role of autophagy in the placenta as a regulator of cell death. Clinical and Experimental Reproductive Medicine. 2014;**41**:97-107. DOI: 10.5653/cerm.2014.41.3.97

[40] Kuma A, Hatano M, Matsui M, Yamamoto A, Nakaya H, Yoshimori T, et al. The role of autophagy during the early neonatal starvation period. Nature. 2004;**432**:1032-1036. DOI: 10.1038/nature03029

[41] Gong GU, Hu L, Liu Y, Bai S, Dai X. Upregulation of HIF-1 α protein induces mitochondrial autophagy in primary cortical cell cultures through the inhibition of the mTOR pathway. International Journal of Molecular Medicine. 2014;**34**:1133-1140. DOI: 10.3892/ijmm.2014.1850

[42] Hung TH, Hsieh TTA, Chen SF, Li MJ, Yeh YL. Autophagy in the human placenta throughout gestation. PLoS One. 2013;**8**:1-11. DOI: 10.1371/journal.pone.0083475

[43] Moscat J, Diaz-Meco MT. p62 at the crossroads of autophagy, apoptosis, and cancer. Cell. 2009;**137**:1001-1004. DOI: 10.1016/j.cell.2009.05.023

[44] Yuk J, Jo E. Crosstalk between autophagy and Inflammasomes. Molecules and Cells. 2013;**36**:393-399. DOI: 10.1007/s10059-013-0298-0

[45] Deretic V. Autophagy: An emerging immunological paradigm. Journal of Immunology. 2012;**189**:15-20. DOI: 10.4049/jimmunol.1102108

[46] Arroyo DS, Gaviglio EA, Ramos JMP, Bussi C, Rodriguez-galan MC, Iribarren P. Autophagy in inflammation, infection, neurodegeneration and cancer. International Immunopharmacology. 2014;**18**:55-65. DOI: 10.1016/j.intimp.2013.11.001

[47] Bauernfeind F, Horvath G, Stutz A, Alnemri ES, Speert D, Fernandes-alnemri T, et al. Cutting edge: NF-kappaB activating pattern recognition and cytokine receptors license NLRP3 inflammasome activation by regulating NLRP3 expression. Journal of Immunology. 2009;**183**(2):787-791. DOI: 10.4049/jimmunol.0901363

[48] Chen GY, Nuñez G. Sterile inflammation: Sensing and reacting to damage. Nature Reviews. Immunology. 2010;**10**(12):826-837. DOI: 10.1038/nri2873

[49] Dupont N, Jiang S, Pilli M, Ornatowski W, Bhattacharya D, Deretic V. Autophagy-based unconventional secretory pathway for extracellular delivery of IL-1 b. The EMBO Journal. 2011;**30**:4701-4711. DOI: 10.1038/emboj.2011.398

[50] Byrne BG, Dubuisson JF, Joshi AD, Persson JJ, Swanson MS. Inflammasome components coordinate autophagy and pyroptosis as macrophage responses to infection. MBio. 2013;**4**(1):e00620-e00612. DOI: 10.1128/mBio.00620-12

[51] Saitoh T, Fujita N, Jang MH, Uematsu S, Yang B-G, Satoh T, et al. Loss of the autophagy protein Atg16L1 enhances endotoxin-induced IL-1beta production. Nature. 2008;**456**:264-268. DOI: 10.1038/nature07383

[52] Martins JD, Liberal J, Silva A, Ferreira I, Neves BM, Cruz MT. Autophagy and inflammasome interplay. DNA and Cell Biology. 2015;**34**:150310073853004. DOI: 10.1089/dna.2014.2752

[53] Nunes PR, Peracoli MTS, Romao-Veiga M, Matias ML, Ribeiro VR, Da Costa Fernandes CJ, et al. Hydrogen peroxide-mediated oxidative stress induces inflammasome activation in term human placental explants. Pregnancy Hypertension. 2018;**14**:29-36. DOI: 10.1016/j.preghy.2018.07.006

[54] Martinon F. Signaling by ROS drives inflammasome activation. European Journal of Immunology. 2010;**40**(3):616-619. DOI: 10.1002/eji.200940168

[55] Lamkanfi M, Vande L, Walle L, Kanneganti TD. Deregulated inflammasome signaling in disease. Immunological Reviews. 2011;**243**(1):163-173. DOI: 10.1111/j.1600-065X.2011.01042.x

[56] Lin X, Li S, Zhao Y, Zhang K, He X, Wang Z. Interaction domains of p62: A bridge between p62 and selective autophagy. DNA and Cell Biology. 2013;**32**(5):220-227. DOI: 10.1089/dna.2012.1915

[57] Harris J. Autophagy and cytokines. Cytokine. 2011;**56**:140-144. DOI: 10.1016/j.cyto.2011.08.022

[58] Hutabarat M, Wibowo N, Obermayer-Pietsch B, Huppertz B. Impact of vitamin D and vitamin D receptor on the trophoblast survival capacity in preeclampsia. PLoS One. 2018;**8**(13):11, e0206725. DOI: 10.1371/journal.pone.0206725. eCollection 2018

[59] Bujold E, Hyett J. Calcium supplementation for prevention of pre-eclampsia. Lancet. 2019;**393**(10169):298-300. DOI: 10.1016/S0140-6736(18)32161-5

[60] Romero R, Garite TJ. Unexpected results of an important trial of vitamins C and E administration to prevent preeclampsia. American Journal of Obstetrics and Gynecology. 2006;**194**(5):1213-1214

[61] Roberts JM, Speer P. Antioxidant therapy to prevent preeclampsia. Seminars in Nephrology. 2004;**24**(6):557-564

[62] Zou Y, Zuo Q, Huang S, Yu Z, Jiang Z, Zou S, et al. Resveratrol inhibits trophoblast apoptosis through oxidative stress in preeclampsia-model rats. Molecules. 2014;**19**(12):20570-20579. DOI: 10.3390/molecules191220570

[63] Yu J, Feng L, Hu Y, Zhou Y. Effects of SAC on oxidative stress and NO availability in placenta: potential benefits to preeclampsia. Placenta. 2012;**33**:487-494

[64] Matias ML et al. Endogenous and uric acid-induced activation of NLRP3 inflammasome in pregnant women with preeclampsia. PLoS One. 2015;**10**:e0129095

[65] Larionov A, Krause A, Miller W. A standard curve based method for relative real time PCR data processing. BMC Bioinformatics. 2005;**6**:62. DOI: 10.1186/1471-2105-6-62

Chapter 6

Alteration in Zeta Potential of Erythrocytes in Preeclampsia Patients

Megha N. Karemore and Jasmine G. Avari

Abstract

Erythrocyte is one of the earliest and extensively analyzed blood cells in blood physiological and clinical studies. The erythrocyte membrane is negatively charged and sialic acid residues are responsible for most of the negative charge at the cell surface. This negative charge on the red blood cells (RBC) surface is believed to prevent RBC aggregation. This charge varies in different disease condition which can be determined by zeta potential (ZP) values. The present study deals with alteration in zeta potential of erythrocytes in preeclampsia patients. The mean erythrocytic ZP of control pregnant women taken during third trimester was found to be 21.64 ± 0.3122 mV whereas; when erythrocytic ZP of preeclampsia patients was measured it was found to be 15.13 ± 0.1393 mV which was significantly less than that of control pregnant volunteers. Alteration in zeta potential value was accompanied by endothelial damage which is able to mechanically deform and hemolyze erythrocytes as they pass through the capillaries. It was also observed from determination of lipid peroxidation of erythrocytes, that there is formation of higher concentration of malondialdehyde within the erythrocytes of preeclampsia patients. The data suggest that, in preeclampsia there is excessive accumulation of oxidative stress which causes injury to vascular endothelial cells by generation of lipid peroxides and detachment of sialic acid residues. As a result there is alteration in the net negative surface charge on RBCs extracellular membrane which leads to alteration in zeta potential value. Thus it can be concluded that zeta potential value of erythrocytes can act as a screening test to anticipate pregnancies at high risk for this complication.

Keywords: zeta potential, preeclampsia, erythrocytes, sialic acid, lipid peroxidation, endothelial damage

1. Introduction

Preeclampsia, first described more than 100 years ago, is a major complication of pregnancy, and is associated with increased maternal and fetal mortality and morbidity [1]. It is a hypertensive disorder of human as well as primate pregnancy characterized by a generalized inflammatory state and endothelial dysfunction, resulting in disseminated microangiopathic disease with vasospasm and hypercoagulation [2]. It occurs in 5–7% of all pregnancies and is a leading cause of maternal and fetal morbidity and mortality [3] together with bleeding and infection. Preeclampsia places the mother at risk of convulsions (eclampsia), kidney failure, liver failure and death [4]. Clinically, preeclampsia is defined as hypertension (blood pressure ≥ 140/90 mmHg) and proteinuria (urinary protein ≥ 300 mg/24 h). It is also associated with pathological edema, coagulation abnormalities and decreased uteroplacental blood flow [5–7]. Despite numerous basic, clinical and epidemiologic studies that have been conducted over the past half-century [8], there is no reliable test to identify women at risk for developing this disorder, thus it is important to develop a predictive screening test early in pregnancy so that we can anticipate pregnancies at high risk for this complication [9]. Recently there is a growing interest in characterizing RBC membrane defects in several diseases, as changes in membrane structure contribute to the pathophysiology of the disease process [10].

The cell-surface charge is the key biophysical parameter that depends on the composition of the cytoplasmic membrane and the physiological condition of cells. The general picture of the membrane structure of erythrocyte is that of 'Bilayer lipid membrane' based on the Gorter-Grendel bimolecular leaflet model with a thickness of about 100 Å. The N- and C-terminal segments of 'Glycophorin', the major glycoprotein that spans the RBC membrane may contribute to the surface charge. From an electrophoretic point of view, the human erythrocyte behaves as a 'macropolyanion'. The dominant ionogenic species is the carboxyl group of N-acetyl neuraminic acid or sialic acid. Other ionic components which are involved in charge contribution are the acidic and basic groups of amino acids of proteins [11]. When such a charged particle suspended in a liquid is placed in an electric field, electrophoresis migrates it towards the oppositely charged electrode [12]. This migration is calculated as velocity or mobility of erythrocyte which is used to calculate zeta potential.

Zeta potential is an electrochemical property of cell surfaces that is determined by the net electrical charge of molecules exposed at the surface of cell membranes [13]. So long as the zeta potential of the system remains constant, the fluidity of the system also remains constant. But if the ZP of the system is lowered then the stability of the system undergoes progressive changes [10]. A number of reports indicate that blood levels of lipid peroxidation products are elevated in women with preeclampsia relative to normal pregnancy [14]. It is also associated with oxidative stress and is responsible for the production of reactive oxygen species (ROS) which are the contributory factors for vascular endothelial cell dysfunctioning [15]. Injury to endothelial cell leads to activation of the clotting cascade and promotes platelet aggregation and clot formation [16] which is able to mechanically deform and hemolyze erythrocytes as they pass through the capillaries [17]. A substantial amount of evidence demonstrates that red cell aggregation increases in preeclampsia compared with normotensive pregnant women [18, 19]. Given the effect of endothelial cell injury and red cell aggregation, the purpose of this chapter is to study the effects of the alteration in erythrocytic zeta potential in preeclampsia patients as assessed by the cell electrophoresis technique using zeta-meter system 4.0.

The following materials are required to study the zeta potential, dextrose (Merck), distilled water, lancet, rectified spirit, zeta meter system 4.0. Blood was collected from voluntary donors with preeclampsia (n = 88) and control pregnant women (n = 60) under treatment in Dalvi memorial hospital and Daga memorial hospital, Nagpur. None of the subjects (both control and patients) were addicted to any drug/smoking. Each volunteer provided written consent for the study of their blood sample.

2. Preparation of isotonic dextrose solution

A 5% w/v dextrose solution was prepared by dissolving 5 g of anhydrous dextrose (Merck) in 100 ml of distilled water.

3. Preparation of blood suspension for zeta potential measurement

Approximately 0.01 ml blood is transferred into 50 ml of freshly prepared isotonic dextrose solution. Mean values of the 10 readings are used to calculate the zeta potential according to the basic Helmholtz-Smoluchowski equation as follows:

$$\text{Zeta potential}, \zeta = \frac{4\pi \times V_t \times EM}{D_t}. \quad (1)$$

where V_t = Viscosity of suspending liquid in poises at temperature 't', EM = Electrophoretic mobility at actual temperature, D_t = Dielectric constant, ZP = Voltage in electrostatic units.

4. Estimation of zeta potential of prepared blood sample by zeta meter system 4.0

The zeta potential of the RBCs was is measured using zeta meter system 4.0. Zeta potential is purely an electro kinetic property of the electrical double layer surrounding the system but not the surface of the system itself. The value of zeta potential gives an indication about the stability of the system under study. This quantity is measured by determining the mobility/velocity of the particle under an applied electric field. The value of zeta potential can be obtained from the equation given by Helmholtz-Smoluchowski.

$$\zeta_d = (4\pi\eta/\epsilon)\, V \quad (2)$$

where ζ_d = electro kinetic potential/zeta potential, η = viscosity of dispersion medium, ϵ = dielectric constant of the dispersion medium, V = v/E (mobility of the particle), v = velocity of the particle in cm/s, E = potential gradient in V/cm [20].

A special capillary cell called electrophoretic cell is used for the measurement of zeta potential. The capillary is embedded inside a chamber having electrodes at either of the two ends. Sample is placed from any one end of the electrophoretic cell and electrodes are connected to the cell and electric field at specific voltage is applied (200 V). Charged particles move towards oppositely charged electrode and their velocity is measured and expressed in terms of electro kinetic potential/zeta potential which indicates the mobility of particle under applied electric field. Recently this method is widely used for determining the membrane potential of biological membranes.

In this experiment, fresh capillary blood samples were obtained from volunteer by puncturing the skin with a lancet and blood suspension was prepared as described in above procedure. Prior to zeta potential measurement temperature of the RBC suspensions were measured and detection parameters for ZP measurements such as light intensity, focal plane and tracking duration were optimized for stable data collection. The RBC suspensions were then added to the previously cleaned and calibrated (using min-u-sil) zeta-meter cell placed under the zeta-meter stage and the mobility of individual RBCs was tracked by equipped

Zeta meter-ZM4DAQ software using microscopically-acquired video images, and data were recorded 10 times for each sample and average zeta-potential in mv was determined using a standard Helmholtz-Smoluchowski formula.

5. Result

The results of blood samples obtained from both patients and control are expressed as mean values with standard deviation. Comparison between different groups and interpretation of results are based on 'two-sample t test' with software PRISM 5. Differences between the groups were considered significant at $p < 0.05$ which indicates that the control and other patient groups differ significantly from one another in all situations. The ZP of erythrocytes was measured by the cell electrophoresis technique using zeta meter system 4.0 at the minimum voltage required for the movement of the erythrocytes to travel a fixed distance. In a study conducted in India, **Table 1** shows the zeta potential (ZP) values of the erythrocytes of control pregnant women in mV while **Table 2** shows the zeta potential (ZP) values erythrocytes of preeclampsia patients in mV [21] (reference of your work). The mean erythrocytic ZP of control pregnant women taken during third trimester was found to be 21.64 ± 0.3122 mV whereas; when erythrocytic ZP of preeclampsia patients was measured it was found to be 15.13 ± 0.1393 mV. The results as shown in **Figure 1** revealed that there is a significant decrease in the ZP of the RBC of preeclampsia patients as compared with the control pregnant women.

Sr. No.	Zeta potential	Sr. No.	Zeta potential	Sr. No.	Zeta potential
1	−23.02 (1.95)	22	−26.28 (1.1)	43	−21.36 (1.41)
2	−21.87 (1.4)	23	−24.07 (1.94)	44	−18.13 (1.6)
3	−17.43 (1.33)	24	−19.34 (0.88)	45	−18.46 (1.98)
4	−24.52 (2.6)	25	−16.82 (0.64)	46	−18.11 (1.69)
5	−19.71 (0.77)	26	−19.52 (1.92)	47	−18.04 (0.84)
6	−22.46 (0.92)	27	−19.02 (2.04)	48	−16.38 (0.83)
7	−16.59 (0.64)	28	−19.83 (1.87)	49	−16.41 (2.5)
8	−20.10 (1.39)	29	−21.26 (0.67)	50	−19.88 (1.7)
9	−24.49 (2.36)	30	−19.62 (1.46)	51	−21.15 (1.03)
10	−21.07 (2.28)	31	−20.73 (1.12)	52	−20.52 (0.84)
11	−17.27 (3.59)	32	−20.11 (0.57)	53	−21.02 (2.76)
12	−24.49 (0.93)	33	−25.59 (1.57)	54	−22.68 (1.79)
13	−21.54 (1.71)	34	−20.57 (0.88)	55	−22.50 (1.2)
14	−26.78 (0.99)	35	−25.73 (1.9)	56	−25.21 (2.15)
15	−19.39 (2.47)	36	−21.68 (1.63)	57	−25.11 (2.77)
16	−22.44 (1.12)	37	−21.13 (1.6)	58	−24.19 (2.28)
17	−20.48 (1.62)	38	−19.68 (1.81)	59	−18.43 (0.77)
18	−20.50 (0.83)	39	−19.96 (1.61)	60	−19.34 (2.75)
19	−23.15 (1.54)	40	−20.75 (1.63)		
20	−21.06 (1.44)	41	-20.36 (2.43)		
21	-21.42 (1.43)	42	-25.65 (1.23)		

Table 1.
Zeta potential of normal pregnant women [21].

Sr. No.	Zeta potential	Sr. No.	Zeta potential	Sr. No.	Zeta potential	Sr. No.	Zeta potential
1	−16.00 (1.42)	23	−16.00 (0.94)	45	−15.62 (0.93)	67	−16.75 (1.62)
2	−13.94 (0.4)	24	−16.16 (0.87)	46	−12.91 (1.58)	68	−14.13 (0.27)
3	−14.45 (0.29)	25	−14.67 (0.8)	47	−15.99 (1.15)	69	−16.5 (1.21)
4	−16.7 (2.1)	26	−15.53 (1.08)	48	−14.94 (0.68)	70	−16.41 (2.5)
5	−14.68 (1.21)	27	−16.74 (2.27)	49	−14.02 (0.35)	71	−15.27 (1.18)
6	−14.00 (0.71)	28	−16.84 (1.12)	50	−16.58 (0.77)	72	−14.28 (0.57)
7	−16.81 (1.03)	29	−16.53 (1.74)	51	−16.14 (0.57)	73	−13.39 (0.34)
8	−13.44 (0.68)	30	−16.49 (1.12)	52	−15.92 (1.35)	74	−16.07 (0.43)
9	−14.75 (0.4)	31	−14.38 (1.12)	53	−16.68 (1.11)	75	−14.28 (0.4)
10	−15.59 (1.11)	32	−13.71 (0.48)	54	−14.07 (0.73)	76	−13.82 (1.86)
11	−15.51 (1.09)	33	−14.86 (0.85)	55	−14.07 (0.95)	77	−16.71 (1.44)
12	−16.14 (1.52)	34	−16.24 (1.15)	56	−12.13 (0.67)	78	−14.38 (1.12)
13	−12.08 (1.08)	35	−15.24 (1.67)	57	−13.55 (0.62)	79	−14.81 (0.55)
14	−16.59 (0.64)	36	−16.59 (0.89)	58	−16.59 (0.22)	80	−15.32 (0.34)
15	−16.45 (0.73)	37	−14.1 (0.57)	59	−16.89 (0.58)	81	−16.38 (0.83)
16	−14.61 (1.79)	38	−13.86 (1.28)	60	−14.96 (1.26)	82	−13.72 (0.83)
17	−12.12 (0.39)	39	−12.42 (0.83)	61	−16.77 (0.42)	83	−13.72 (2.36)
18	−15.87 (2.1)	40	−13.86 (0.82)	62	−15.28 (0.36)	84	−16.28 (0.94)
19	−15.18 (1.1)	41	−16.92 (1.74)	63	−16.52 (1.32)	85	−12.05 (1.05)
20	−13.72 (0.83)	42	−15.61 (1.08)	64	−15.44 (0.6)	86	−14.65 (0.6)
21	−13.52 (0.48)	43	−13.55 (0.62)	65	−14.81 (1.52)	87	−16.72 (0.46)
22	−16.83 (1.08)	44	−14.67 (0.8)	66	−16.82 (0.64)	88	−13.82 (1.86)

Table 2.
Zeta potential of preeclampsia patients [21].

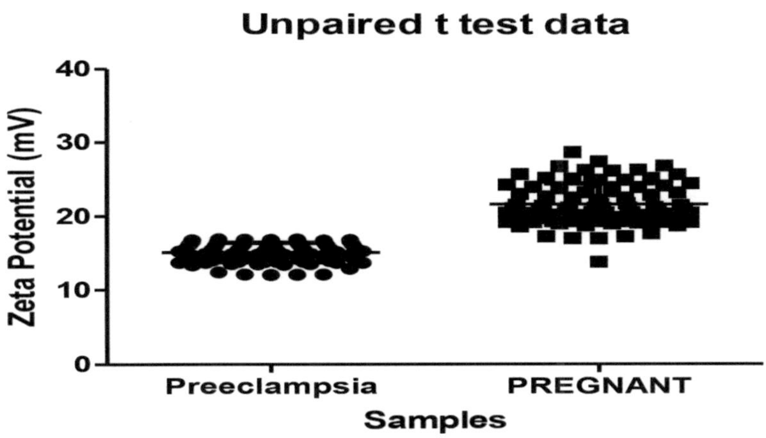

Figure 1.
Comparison of erythrocytic zeta potential of preeclampsia patients and control pregnant women [21].

6. Discussion

Zeta potential (ZP) is an electrochemical property of cell surfaces that is determined by the net electrical charge of molecules exposed at the surface of cell membranes. Membrane proteins contribute to the total net electrical charge of cell surfaces and can alter ZP through changes in their intermolecular interactions [22]. Erythrocyte is one of the earliest and extensively analyzed blood cells in blood physiological and clinical studies [23]. The erythrocyte membrane is negatively charged and the major contributor to the negative ZP of RBCs is sialic acid, which is abundantly present on the RBC surface [24, 25]. This negative charge on the RBC surface is believed to prevent RBC aggregation [25]. The physiologic changes during normal pregnancy affect red cell aggregation [26]. The aggregation properties of the cells depend, in turn, on the shape and concentration of red blood cells (RBCs) as well as the presence of sticky proteins [27]. In a cross-sectional study, Ozanne et al. demonstrated that red cells aggregation increases during the course of normal pregnancy [28]. Whereas, in preeclampsia red blood cell aggregation is further increased when compared with normotensive pregnant women; this increase could be due to either the changes in fibrinogen system or functional abnormalities of erythrocyte membranes [22]. Andrea et al. observed that erythrocyte aggregation was increased in all the hypertensive pregnant patients compared with the normotensive pregnant controls, regardless of both the onset (chronic or pregnancy-induced) of hypertension and the status of plasma macromolecules. Thus, concluded that increased erythrocyte aggregation may be due to either conformational changes of the membrane occurring during hypertension or a redistribution of the ionic charges on the two surfaces of the membrane [23]. The membrane zeta potential and the morphology are the important structural and functional parameters of erythrocytes. They affect the deformability and the circulation of erythrocytes in a blood vessel. On the other hand, they influence the affinity, aggregation, metabolism and immunity of the cell [25]. Accordingly, in this study, we performed systematic measurements of the membrane zeta potential during preeclampsia and comparison was done between blood samples from pregnant women as control vs. preeclampsia patients.

7. Conclusion

The zeta potential values of the erythrocytes of pregnant women and preeclampsia patients were determined by cell electrophoresis technique using zeta meter system 4.0. Zeta potential (ZP) is a characteristic signature for the diagnosis of hemolytic diseases, studies of membrane permeability, and alterations leading to destruction of erythrocytes. To investigate the properties of the erythrocyte membrane, we examined the zeta potential measurements for the surfaces of erythrocyte of preeclampsia patients during each trimester. The electrochemical potential value obtained for preeclampsia patient erythrocytes was found to be reduced in comparison with the normal pregnant women erythrocyte. Thus it is concluded that increased erythrocyte aggregation may be due to either conformational changes of the membrane occurring during hypertension or a redistribution of the ionic charges on the two surfaces of the membrane and hence reduces the zeta potential of preeclampsia patients' erythrocytes. Measurement of zeta potential is an easy and relatively quick way to detect molecular changes that have occurred on the membrane surface of erythrocytes.

Acknowledgements

The authors would like to thank Dalvi memorial hospital and research center, Nagpur and Daga memorial hospital, Nagpur for their support during the research work.

Author details

Megha N. Karemore* and Jasmine G. Avari
Department of Pharmaceutical Sciences, R. T. M. Nagpur University, Nagpur, Maharashtra, India

*Address all correspondence to: meghakaremore0687@gmail.com

References

[1] Garner PR, D'Alton ME, Dudley DK, Huard P, Hardie M. Preeclampsia in diabetic pregnancies. American Journal of Obstetrics and Gynecology. 1990;**163**(2):505-508

[2] Ness RB, Roberts JM. Heterogeneous causes constituting the single syndrome of preeclampsia: A hypothesis and its implications. American Journal of Obstetrics and Gynecology. 1996;**175**:1365-1370

[3] Cunningham FG et al. Williams Obstetrics. New York, USA: McGraw-Hill; 2001

[4] Roberts JM et al. Summary of the NHLBI working group on research on hypertension during pregnancy. Hypertension. 2003;**41**:437-445

[5] Chavarria ME et al. Prostacyclin/thromboxane early changes in pregnancies that are complicated by preeclampsia. American Journal of Obstetrics and Gynecology. 2003;**188**:986-992

[6] Walsh SW. Eicosanoids in preeclampsia. Prostaglandins, Leukotrienes, and Essential Fatty Acids. 2004;**70**:223-232

[7] Gervasi MT et al. Phenotypic and metabolic characteristics of monocytes and granulocytes in preeclampsia. American Journal of Obstetrics and Gynecology. 2001;**185**:792-797

[8] Roccella EJ. National high blood pressure education program working group report on high blood pressure in pregnancy. Consensus report. American Journal of Obstetrics and Gynecology. 1990;**163**:1689-1712

[9] Davari Tanha F, Mohammad Pour J, Kaveh M, Shariat M. Prediction of preeclampsia with elevation in erythroblast count in maternal blood. Shiraz E Medical Journal. 2008;**9**(3):120-128

[10] Adak S, Chowdhury S, Bhattacharyya M. Dynamic and electro kinetic behaviour of erythrocyte membrane in diabetes mellitus and diabetic cardiovascular disease. Biochimica et Biophysica Acta. 2008;**1780**:108-115

[11] Dungore JR. Studies on electrokinetic potential of erythrocytes during pregnancy and related pathological conditions [PhD dissertation]. Nagpur: Nagpur University; 1988. pp. 9-11

[12] Becher P. Emulsions Theory and Practice. New York: Reinhold; 1965

[13] Tokumasu F, Ostera GR, Amaratunga C, Fairhurst RM. Modifications in erythrocyte membrane zeta potential by plasmodium falciparum infection. Experimental Parasitology. 2012;**131**:245-251

[14] Hubel CA et al. Lipid peroxidation in pregnancy: New perspectives on preeclampsia. American Journal of Obstetrics and Gynecology. 1989;**161**:1025-1034

[15] Walsh SW. Obesity: A risk factor for preeclampsia. Trends in Endocrinology and Metabolism. 2007;**18**(10):365-370

[16] Roberts JM et al. Preeclampsia: An endothelial cell disorder. American Journal of Obstetrics and Gynecology. 1989;**161**:1200-1204

[17] Hernandez Hernandez JD et al. Morphological changes of red blood cells in peripheral blood smear of patients with pregnancy-related hypertensive disorders. Archives of Medical Research. 2015;**46**:479-483

[18] Gamzu R et al. Increased erythrocyte adhesiveness and aggregation in peripheral venous blood of women with pregnancy-induced hypertension. Obstetrics and Gynecology. 2001;**98**:307-312

[19] Ozanne P, Linderkamp O, Millerand FC, Meiselman HJ. Erythrocyte aggregation during normal pregnancy. American Journal of Obstetrics and Gynecology. 1983;**147**:576

[20] Becher P. Emulsions, Theory and Practice. 2nd ed. New York: Reinhold; 1965

[21] Karemore MN, Avari JG. Zeta potential as a novel diagnostic tool for preeclampsia. Pregnancy Hypertension. 2018;**13**:187-197

[22] Tranquilli AL, Mazzanti L, Bertoli E, Romanini C. Sodium/potassium adenosine triphosphatase on erythrocyte ghosts from pregnant women and its relationship to pregnancy-induced hypertension. Obstetrics and Gynecology. 1988;**74**:627-630

[23] Tranquilli AL et al. Nifedipine treatment in preeclampsia reverts the increased erythrocyte aggregation to normal. American Journal of Obstetrics and Gynecology. 1992;**167**:942-945

[24] Jorge DH et al. Morphological changes of red blood cells in peripheral blood smear of patients with pregnancy-related hypertensive disorders. Archives of Medical Research. 2015;**46**:479-483

[25] Chen X-Y, Huang Y-X, Liu W-j, Yuan Z-j. Membrane surface charge and morphological and mechanical properties of young and old erythrocytes. Current Applied Physics. 2007;**7**(S1):e94-e96

[26] Gamzu R et al. Increased erythrocyte adhesiveness and aggregation in peripheral venous blood of women with pregnancy-induced hypertension. American Journal of Obstetrics and Gynecology. 2001;**98**:307-312

[27] Chien S. Biophysical behavior of red cells in suspension. In: Surgenor D, editor. The Red Blood Cell. Vol. 2. New York: Academic Press; 1975. p. 1031

[28] Ozanne P, Linderkamp O, Miller FC, Meiselman HJ. Erythrocyte aggregation during normal pregnancy. American Journal of Obstetrics and Gynecology. 1983;**147**:576-583

Chapter 7

Biochemical Dysregulation of Pre-Eclampsia and Gestational Diabetes Mellitus

Maria Portelli and Byron Baron

Abstract

Emerging evidence indicates that among the various pregnancy complications, pre-eclampsia and gestational diabetes mellitus (GDM) seem to have, at least in part, shared underlying ethiologies. Apart from sharing numerous risk factors, it has been shown that the rate of pre-eclampsia is influenced by the presence and severity of GDM, with hyperglycemia due to insulin resistance and the biochemical changes this brings about (angiogenic imbalance, oxidative stress and inflammation), playing some role in the pathogenesis of endothelial dysfunction leading to the development of pre-eclampsia. However, so far the biochemical mechanisms underlying and linking these two conditions is still not properly understood. The altered physiological parameters, dysregulation of potential protein biomarkers and DNA-related changes (mutations, methylations, miRNAs) will be combined in this review to explore possible underlying mechanisms.

Keywords: pre-eclampsia, gestational diabetes mellitus, endothelial dysfunction, insulin resistance, angiogenic factors, oxidative stress, inflammation

Key points

- A combination of maternal risk factors appears to contribute to the similar biochemical dysregulation present in both pre-eclampsia and GDM.
- The common biochemical characteristics underlying these conditions include endothelial dysfunction, angiogenic imbalance, insulin resistance, oxidative stress, inflammation and dyslipidemia.
- Detailed evaluation of pre-pregnancy characteristics and clearer distinction between the different disease statuses is required to better understand the shared and separate biochemical pathways.

1. Pathophysiology of pre-eclampsia and gestational diabetes mellitus

Pre-eclampsia is a multisystem, pregnancy-specific disorder, presenting new-onset hypertension and proteinuria after 20 weeks of gestation. It is a leading cause of maternal and foetal morbidity and mortality, with delivery being the only known cure. Pre-eclampsia complicates 2–5% of pregnancies in Europe and America and can reach up to 10% of pregnancies in developing countries [1].

Pre-eclampsia is characterised by a first, asymptomatic stage involving impaired trophoblastic penetration of the decidua (both into the superficial myometrium at 14–16 weeks and into the deep myometrium at 18–20 weeks), limiting the remodelling of the maternal uterine spiral arteries for uteroplacental blood perfusion and producing local placental hypoxia and oxidative stress, which consequently leads to insufficient blood perfusion, inflammation, apoptosis, and structural damage. In the second stage, placental factors released into the maternal circulation from the poorly perfused placenta, together with the aberrant expression of pro-inflammatory, anti-angiogenic, and angiogenic factors, eventually cause the endothelial dysfunction that leads to the main clinical symptoms of pre-eclampsia [1].

This disorder can have an early onset (before 34 weeks of gestation) or a late onset (after 34 weeks of gestation), with the placentas of women with early onset pre-eclampsia presenting hypoplasia (small placental size) and a significantly higher number of placental vascular lesions compared to those with late onset PE, which present hyperplasia (increased placental size) and histological evidence of placental inflammation, with absence of vascular insufficiency, suggesting that pre-eclampsia might be more than a single condition [2].

Gestational diabetes mellitus (GDM) is defined as hyperglycemia that is first diagnosed during pregnancy. This definition of GDM does not preclude the possible existence of unrecognised pre-pregnancy diabetes. The prevalence of GDM ranges from 2 to 10% of all pregnancies in developed countries [3] and is associated with birth complications, including macrosomia and operative delivery. GDM develops from a dysfunction of the pancreatic Beta cells such that the insulin supply is inadequate to meet tissue demands for normal blood glucose regulation. This insulin resistance leads to increased levels of glucose production and free fatty acids, with subsequent increased blood glucose levels [4].

All forms of diabetes (GDM, type 1 diabetes - T1D and type 2 diabetes mellitus - T2DM) increase the risk of pre-eclampsia, with GDM being an independent risk factor for the development of pre-eclampsia [5, 6], and pre-existing diabetes being a risk factor for both early- and late-onset pre-eclampsia [7]. The incidence of pre-eclampsia increases from 2–7% of pregnancies in non-diabetic women to 15–20% in women with T1D and 10–14% in women with T2DM [8].

Pre-eclampsia and GDM share a number of risk factors, including advanced maternal age, nulliparity, multifetal pregnancies, non-white ethnicity, and pre-pregnancy obesity [5, 9]. Both pre-eclampsia and GDM also have long-term health implications, with pre-eclampsia increasing the risk of future cardiovascular disease, stroke, kidney disease, ophthalmic disease and development of T2DM (even without GDM), while GDM increases the risk of cardiovascular disease and T2DM for both mother and child [8].

Although the exact pathophysiology is still unknown, it would seem that a combination of maternal risk factors contribute to the similar biochemical dysregulation present in both pre-eclampsia and GDM, compared to healthy pregnancies, including endothelial dysfunction, angiogenic imbalance, insulin resistance, oxidative stress, inflammation and dyslipidemia [8] suggests shared etiological pathways underlying these conditions. Such biochemical changes might result from a common aetiology, have a common trigger (such as insulin resistance during pregnancy [10]) or be similar responses to different underlying disease processes that existed prior to pregnancy [11]. Similarly, genetic and/or environmental factors that contribute to pre-eclampsia could also increase the risk of diabetic complications later in life or it could be just as possible that pre-eclampsia causes lasting damage that leads to diabetic complications years after pregnancy [8].

2. Endothelial dysfunction

Within the placenta, limited remodelling of the maternal uterine spiral arteries may cause hypoxia [12] or repeated ischemia–reperfusion injury [13], such that the damaged placenta then releases factors into the maternal circulation that contribute to vascular dysfunction [12]. These include the anti-angiogenic proteins soluble vascular endothelial growth factor receptor 1 (sVEGFR-1; or more commonly known as soluble fms-like tyrosine kinase 1 - sFlt-1) and soluble endoglin (sEng) [14, 15]. Excess of these anti-angiogenic proteins contributes to systemic maternal endothelial dysfunction in women with pre-eclampsia [16].

The sFlt-1 protein is a truncated form of VEGF receptor 1, composed of six immunoglobulin-like domains from the ligand-binding, extracellular domain [1]. Once secreted, sFlt-1 binds to the pro-angiogenic ligands vascular endothelial growth factor (VEGF) and placental growth factor (PlGF), acting as a as a non-signalling decoy, reducing their bio-availability and enhancing endothelial dysfunction [16–18].

The sEng protein is composed of the extracellular domain of Endoglin, following proteolytic cleavage by metalloproteinase (MMP)-14. It binds to Transforming Growth Factor-b1 (TGF-β1), inhibiting binding to Endoglin (a TGF-β1 co-receptor), preventing the activation of endothelial Nitric Oxide Synthase (NOS) and subsequent vasodilation [15].

The levels of sFlt-1 and sEng were found to be proportional to the severity of pre-eclampsia [19–21], with maternal plasma concentrations of sFlt-1 and sEng increasing before pre-eclampsia was diagnosed, making them potential biomarkers for the disease [1, 22–29]. Concomitantly, the increase of sFlt-1 brings about a decrease in maternal plasma concentration of PlGF [18, 30–32]. However, the relative change in sFlt1 and sEng concentrations between two consecutive visits (first and second trimester) seems more useful as a predictive marker for developing pre-eclampsia among both low- and high-risk women that the absolute concentrations [30, 33].

The relationship between anti-angiogenic factors and pre-eclampsia in women with GDM has been explored only in a handful of studies. Women with GDM were found to have higher serum sFlt-1, Placental Protein 13 (PP13), Pentraxin 3 (PTX3), myostatin and follistatin levels early in the second trimester, with sFlt-1 and PTX3 having potential predictive value [34]. Quantitative proteomics of syncytiotrophoblasts from women with GDM and pre-eclampsia identified 11 upregulated and 12 downregulated proteins including increased Flt-1 [35]. Moreover, high sEng, high sFlt-1, low PlGF and high sFlt-1/PlGF ratio increased the odds of developing pre-eclampsia among women with pre-existing diabetes [30].

Further vascular dysfunction results from the inhibition of NOS. Asymmetric dimethylarginine (ADMA) is an analogue of L-arginine and endogenous competitive inhibitor of NOS, resulting in reduced NO synthesis from L-arginine and higher superoxide generation. NO is important in maintaining endothelial homeostasis and elevated ADMA levels are associated with inflammation, insulin resistance, dyslipidemia, obesity, and cardiovascular disease. Numerous studies have measured ADMA levels in women with pre-eclampsia and normotensive women but discrepant findings have been observed. Nevertheless, some reported elevated ADMA levels prior to the development of clinical symptoms of PE, which suggests that ADMA may contribute to the pathophysiology of pre-eclampsia [1, 29].

Poor placentation, oxidative stress, endothelial cell dysfunction and altered glucose metabolism among others generate Damage-Associated Molecular Patterns (DAMPs) including Heat Shock Proteins (HSPs), TNF-α, fetal DNA, hyaluronan, oxidised low-density lipoprotein (LDL) and long pentraxin-3 [36]. HSP70 (and its post-translational modifications) has been shown to be elevated in the placentas and sera of women with PE, reflecting systemic inflammation and oxidative stress, with

HSP70 initially protecting against placental oxidative stress but its overexpression may lead to intervillous endothelial dysfunction and may play a role in the pathogenesis of pre-eclampsia [1, 29]. TLR-4 protein expression, which recognises such DAMPs at the feto-maternal interface, is increased in women with pre-eclampsia [37].

3. Insulin resistance

Insulin resistance or hyperinsulinemia is an impaired response to insulin, characteristic of normal pregnancy, which results in increased insulin secretion by the pancreatic β-cells or relative insulin deficiency due to the pancreatic β-cell deterioration. Insulin resistance is due to an overall decreased expression of the insulin receptor substrate (IRS)-1/2 protein, decreased IRS-1/2 tyrosine phosphorylation and increased IRS-1/2 serine phosphorylation, resulting in reduced glucose transport activity, which was found to be even more pronounced in women with pre-eclampsia and GDM, which might also underlie the future risk for developing T2DM [38].

Insulin resistance via the inhibition of IRS1/2 results in impaired activation of the phosphoinositide 3-kinase (PI3K) and Ak strain transforming (Akt)-dependent signalling pathway, and increased activity of the mammalian target of rapamycin (mTOR) resulting from lower activity of the mitogen activated protein kinase (MAPK) pathway. The reduced Akt activity leads to a decreased production of nitric oxide (NO) (a vasodilator) and increase of endothelin (ET)-1 (a vasoconstrictor) [39], linking endothelial dysfunction and increased risk of pre-eclampsia with GDM.

Compared to normotesive women, women who develop pre-eclampsia are more insulin resistant prior to pregnancy [40], in the first and second trimesters [41], and years after pregnancy [42], and in fact a number of pre-eclampsia risk factors are also associated with insulin resistance [40, 41]. The same was found in women that developed GDM, presenting chronic insulin resistance and chronic β-cell function prior to pregnancy [4, 43]. Women with GDM are then unable to increase insulin production to compensate for the increased insulin resistance and destruction, as happens in normal pregnancy [44]. The metabolic changes observed in GDM are the same as those found in the pre-diabetic stages of T2DM, where pre-diabetes may include patients with metabolic syndrome, GDM, and impaired glucose tolerance.

4. Oxidative stress and mitochondrial dysfunction

During normal pregnancy generation of reactive oxygen species (ROS) is known to be increased and necessary for proper physiology [45]. However, both pre-eclampsia and GDM present a reduced antioxidant status when compared to normal pregnancies, with increased levels of protein and lipid oxidation products [46]. Free radicals react with nucleic acids, proteins and lipids, bring about post-translational modification of proteins [47] and cause structural and functional damage [46]. The changes in a wide variety of oxidative stress metabolites (such as NO, superoxide and peroxynitrile) as well as antioxidant enzymes and compounds (such as catalase, superoxide dismutase (SOD) and vitamin E) have been analysed in relation to pre-eclampsia and GDM compared to normal pregnancies but there is still no consensus since their levels were found to be variable (the same, higher or lower) depending on the cohort studied [48–50]. Although supplementation with antioxidants such as vitamin C, vitamin E or n-acetylcysteine have been found to be ineffective in reducing the risk of pre-eclampsia, calcium and vitamin D supplementation could lower risk of pre-eclampsia [50, 51].

In the case of hyperglycemia, it is known to stimulate ROS production by four major sources, namely glucose auto-oxidation, mitochondrial superoxide production, endothelial NOS uncoupling and advanced glycation end product (AGE)-dependent NADPH oxidase activation, with glucose auto-oxidation and mitochondrial superoxide likely being the initial contributors to ROS-mediated dysfunction caused by hyperglycemia [52, 53]. Advanced glycation end products are of particular interest as these were found to be able to promote TNF-α mRNA expression and secretion as well as bringing about a significant decrease in eNOS mRNA expression and protein levels via serine phosphorylation [54, 55].

The serum levels of AGEs were higher in women with both early- and late-onset pre-eclampsia and in women with severe pre-eclampsia positively correlated with serum levels of TNF-α and VCAM-1, indicating AGEs are important mediators in regulating the inflammatory pathways of pre-eclampsia [56–58]. Furthermore, treatment with AGEs increased intracellular ROS generation and over-expression of sFlt-1 in an extravillous trophoblast cell line, suggesting that AGEs may be important mediators in the regulation of angiogenic pathways, with accumulation of AGEs possibly contributing to pre-eclampsia by promoting sFlt-1 production via the activation of a RAGE/NADPH oxidase dependent pathway [59].

In women with PE, oxidative markers were significantly higher, while anti-oxidative markers were significantly lower, indicating gradual oxidative damage of the placenta, even before the onset of clinical symptoms [60]. Similarly, women with GDM had higher serum malondialdehyde levels and significantly lower serum glutathione peroxidase activity in the first trimester, with negative correlation in the second and third trimester [61].

Looking directly at the mitochondria, women with early-onset pre-eclampsia showed increased mitochondrial activation, with up-regulation of optic atrophy, type 1 (OPA-1), increased placental mitochondrial DNA copy number, and mitochondrial transcription factor A down-regulation, while both early- and late-onset pre-eclampsia were associated with an elevated phosphate/oxygen ratio [62]. Moreover, a comparative proteomics analysis of placental mitochondria in women with pre-eclampsia compared to healthy pregnancies identified up-regulation of 4 proteins and down-regulation of 22 proteins involved in ROS generation, apoptosis, fatty acid oxidation, respiratory chain function, and the tricarboxylic acid cycle [63].

5. Inflammation

5.1 Cytokines

After ischemia and reperfusion injury, together with oxidative stress, the placenta mounts an inflammatory response releasing cytokines and other inflammatory factors such as Tumour Necrosis Factor-alpha (TNF-α), Interleukin (IL)-6, and C-reactive protein (CRP), and damaging levels of ROS, which are a characteristic of pre-eclampsia [64] and the altered levels of inflammatory cytokines in both early and late-onset pre-eclampsia correlated with the type of histopathologic changes in the placenta [65].

The proposed mechanism linking insulin resistance and inflammatory pathways involves a reduction in Akt activity, which also reduces NO generation. Reduced Akt activity and reduced plasma level of adiponectin reduce adenosine monophosphate protein kinase (AMPK) activity, such that mTOR activation is facilitated. The increased mTOR-activated signalling and increased extracellular level of leptin and TNF-α result in c-Jun N-terminal kinase (JNK) activation, inhibiting IRS1/2 and reducing insulin signalling. Thus hyperinsulinemia activates a feedback loop of increased vascular inflammation and insulin resistance [39].

In women who later developed GDM, increased leukocyte counts were observed since the first trimester, indicating that inflammation is associated with the development of GDM [66]. Women with GDM had higher serum levels of TNF-α in the third trimester and TNF-α and IL-6 at term, compared to women with normoglycemia during pregnancy, and TNF-α levels were inversely correlated with insulin sensitivity [67–69]. Moreover, the increase of TNF-α concentration from pregravid to the third trimester was the best predictor of insulin resistance in pregnancy when compared with leptin, cortisol, and other pregnancy-derived hormones independent of fat mass [67]. Years after pregnancy, women with GDM were still found to have higher circulating levels of the inflammatory mediators CRP, Plasminogen Activator Inhibitor-1 (PAI-1), fibrinogen and IL-6, and lower levels of adiponectin, compared to non-diabetic women, increasing the risk for future development of inflammatory-related conditions [70].

5.2 Adipokines

Adipokines (proteins secreted from adipocytes) are involved in a wide range of physiological processes including haemostasis, lipid metabolism, atherosclerosis, blood pressure regulation, insulin sensitivity, angiogenesis, immunity and inflammation, and have been shown to play a role in normal pregnancy [71].

In both pre-eclampsia and GDM, various adipokines are dysregulated, and could be involved in the pathophysiology of these conditions, especially since obesity is a known risk factor for both [72–74]. The most well-studied are adiponectin and leptin. Adiponectin is considered an insulin-sensitising, anti-inflammatory and anti-atherogenic adipokine, which stimulates glucose uptake in skeletal muscle and reduces hepatic glucose production through AMP-activated protein kinase [75]. Leptin plays a key role in the regulation of energy intake and energy expenditure (increasing insulin sensitivity by influencing insulin secretion, glucose utilisation, glycogen synthesis and fatty acid metabolism) and is involved in a number of physiological processes including regulation of gonadotrophin-releasing hormone (GnRH) secretion, inflammation, immune response, reproduction and angiogenesis [76].

Increased concentrations of adiponectin were found in women with pre-eclampsia [77–80], which could be a mechanism to counter the inflammatory response and improve insulin sensitivity and vascular function [81]. Inversely, decreased concentrations of adiponectin, and up-regulated expression of its receptor adiponectin receptor-1 (ADIPOR1), were found in women with GDM [82–85], possibly suppressed by TNF-α, other proinflammatory mediators and insulin [38], which might further aggravate insulin resistance since adiponectin has insulin-sensitising effects. Adiponectin levels during pregnancy were also found to predict postpartum insulin sensitivity and ß-cell function, even among non-obese women [86].

High levels of leptin were found both in women with pre-eclampsia [77, 87–89], even before the clinical onset of the disease [90–93] (suggesting a pathophysiological role), and women with GDM [69, 94–96]. In pre-eclampsia pregnancies increased leptin concentrations affect metabolic, immune, and angiogenic responses, regulating placental growth (potentially resulting in placental hypertrophy), stimulating angiogenesis and increased blood supply to the placenta as well as regulating placental nutrient transport, use, and storage of lipids and amino acids, possibly as a compensatory mechanism to increase nutrient delivery to the underperfused placenta [97]. In GDM pregnancies leptin acts as a pro-inflammatory adipokine, being associated with increased production of pro-inflammatory cytokines (IL-6 and TNF-α), stimulating the production of CC-chemokine ligands (CCL3, CCL4 and CCL5), production of ROS and promoting cell proliferation and migratory responses [98].

5.3 Peroxisome proliferator-activated receptors

Peroxisome proliferator-activated receptors (PPARs) are ligand-activated transcription factors that form part of the nuclear hormone receptor superfamily, that regulate genes involved in metabolic, anti-inflammatory and developmental processes. There are three mammalian types of PPARs namely PPARα, PPARβ/δ, and PPARγ. PPARs perform functions throughout pregnancy including implantation, trophoblast differentiation and placental function, and are also involved in embryonic and fetal development. The regulation of metabolic and anti-inflammatory pathways by the PPAR system is considered crucial in the development of GDM [99].

During normal pregnancy, PPARγ activators such as specific prostanoids or fatty acid derivatives are upregulated in maternal serum [100]. In women with PE, circulating PPARγ ligands have been shown to be suppressed even before clinical presentation [101]. Animal models have shown that administration of a PPARγ antagonist early during gestational results in PE-like symptoms (such as elevated blood pressure, proteinuria, endothelial dysfunction, and increased platelet aggregation) [102], while treatment with a PPARγ agonist improves pregnancy outcome in animals with pre-eclampsia by reducing oxidative stress in a heme oxygenase (HO)-1-dependent pathway [103]. Another study found that while the placentas of women with pre-eclampsia did not present any changes PPAR protein expression or DNA binding activity, those from women with GDM presented decreased PPARγ and PPARα protein concentrations and decreased concentrations of RXRα (the heterodimer partner of PPARγ) [104].

6. Genetic and epigenetic influences

6.1 Genetics

Besides the finding that women having their first baby with a family history of pre-eclampsia increases two- to five-fold the risk of developing PE, the genetic predisposition to pre-eclampsia has been studied to various degrees, with genetic factors possibly playing a role in increased sFlt-1 production and placental size, imprinted genes possibly involved in the maternal contribution to develop pre-eclampsia and a number of genetic disorders being associated with pre-eclampsia (trisomy 13, angiotensinogen gene variant T235, eNOS, genes causing thrombophilia, and a number of SNPs) despite little significance [105]. pre-eclampsia is an extremely complex spectrum disorder with gene clusters falling into four categories, those involved in (i) hormone secretion, response to hypoxia, and response to nutrient levels; (ii) immune and inflammatory responses (including cytokine/interferon signalling); (iii) metabolism, cell proliferation and cell cycle as well as stress response and DNA damage; (iv) hormone secretion and ion channel activity, and nervous system development or neurological system processes [106].

A few studied have looked into the genetics of GDM and its genetic relationship with T2DM with the major genes being *MTNR1B, TCF7L2, IRS1, IGF2BP2, TNF-α* and *PPARG* [107, 108]. Genes linked to GDM participate in cell functions involving cell activation, immune response, organ development, and regulation of cell death [109], but do not shed light on the underlying cause of the disorder.

6.2 DNA methylation

The effects of pre-eclampsia and GDM on the intrauterine environment also bring about epigenetic modifications including DNA methylation [110]. Although the placenta is known to be hypomethylated relative to other tissues [111], studies measuring CpG island methylation in the RefSeq genes (i.e. mainly promoter methylation, covering about 1.5% of total genomic CpGs) found a predominance of hypermethylation at methylation variable positions in the placentas of women with pre-eclampsia or GDM, with dysregulation of metabolic pathways, signalling pathways and immune response pathways [112–120]. When interrogating global placental DNA methylation, a preliminary study showed a negative association between the degree of methylation and both pre-eclampsia and GDM [121]. However, a much larger study later found increased placental global DNA hypermethylation in GDM women, independent of other risk factors [122].

One driver for DNA hypermethylation in the placenta might be oxidative stress, since both pre-eclampsia and GDM are associated with increased oxidative stress and it has been shown in a T2DM rat model that this condition brings about global DNA hypermethylation in the liver, and that DNA hypermethylation can be reduced by polyphenols that act as antioxidants [123–125].

6.3 Regulatory microRNAs

The miRNA expression pattern in the placenta (predominantly in the trophoblast) changes throughout pregnancy due to the involvement of miRNAs in regulating different aspects of trophoblast biology [126]. Such changes are also detectable in the maternal plasma [127, 128].

A number of studies have identified over 100 differentially expressed miRNAs in the placenta or sera of women with pre-eclampsia compared to normotensive controls. Among these are miRNAs involved in cellular proliferation, cellular migration, inflammation, signal transduction, vascular remodelling and mitochondrial function [126, 129–134]. Increased plasma levels of miR-210 were associated with the severity of pre-eclampsia [135].

The studies focusing on miRNAs in the sera of women with GDM are fewer as are the identified miRNAs (around 50 in total). The processes that seem to be mostly targeted by miRNAs in GDM are insulin/IGF1 signalling (IRS-1, IRS-2, SOS-1, MAPK-1, Insig1, PCK2), adipogenesis, endothelial function, inflammation (TGF-β signalling pathway), and energy balance (EGFR/PI3K/Akt/mTOR signalling pathway) [136–139]. Moreover, 9 miRNAs were found to be shared among T1D, T2DM and GDM, with an additional 19 miRNAs specific to GDM, indicating that GDM leads to changes that differ from those of the other forms of diabetes [140]. Interestingly, the histone methyltransferase enhancer of zester homologue 2 isoform beta (EZH2-β) has been linked to GDM via miRNA control [141].

7. Insight from metformin

Metformin (1,1-Dimethylbiguanide) is a small molecule that can readily cross the placental barrier [142]. It is the treatment of choice for GDM due to its efficacy and safety for the unborn child compared to insulin [143]. Metformin acts through the mitochondria, by inhibiting complex I of the electron transport chain, activating AMPK that controls cellular energy homeostasis and thus reduces gluconeogenesis and enhanced insulin suppression of endogenous glucose production by the liver [144].

Metformin was shown to be superior to insulin in reducing the frequency of gestational hypertension and possibly pre-eclampsia [145–147], by reducing ROS production, reducing endothelial dysfunction (by reducing sFlt-1 and sEng secretion regulated through the mitochondria), reducing inflammation (by reducing VCAM-1 mRNA expression induced by TNF–α), enhancing vasodilation and inducing angiogenesis [47, 148]. This suggests that there are similar perturbations in the cellular energy balance of patients with pre-eclampsia and GDM.

8. Conclusions

Much of the biochemical dysregulation that is common to both GDM and pre-eclampsia suggests overlapping pathophysiology (**Figure 1**). However, the available data does not clearly outline a common etiologic pathway, mainly due to limited analysis power to compare the different patient groups. Detailed evaluation of pre-pregnancy characteristics and clearer distinction between the different disease

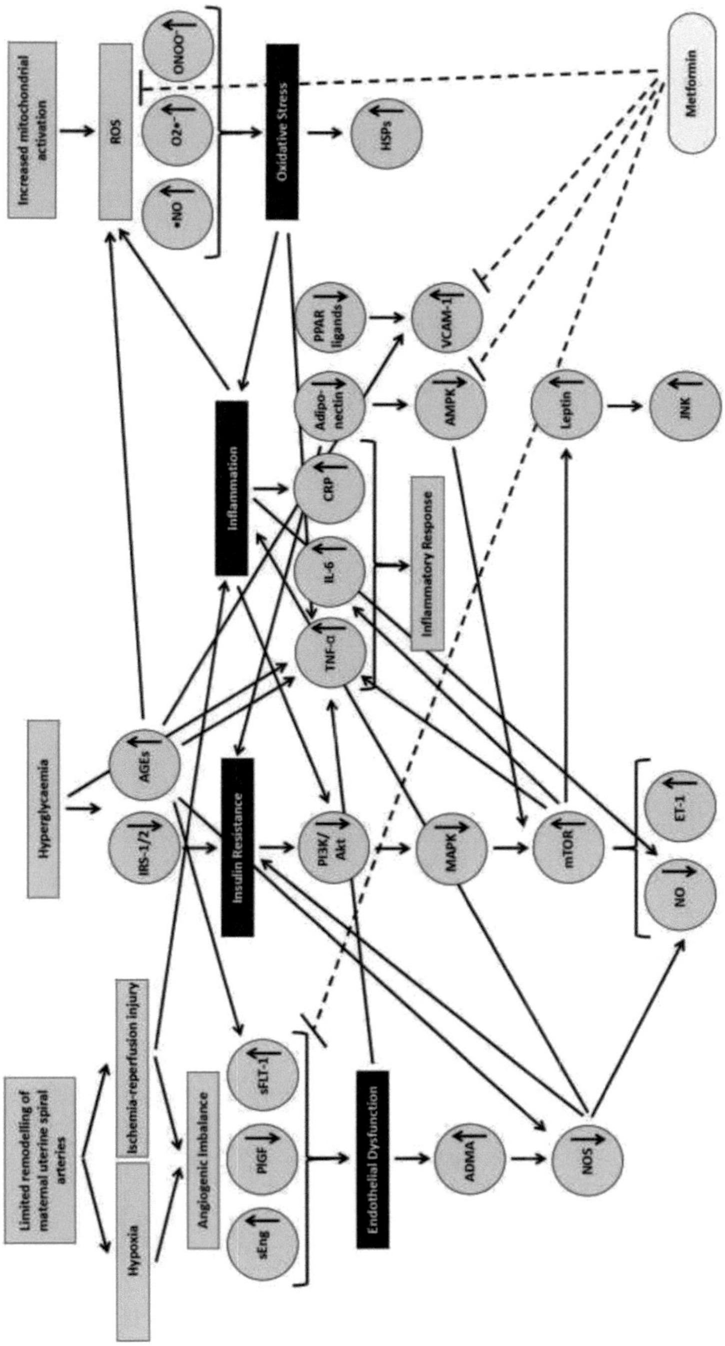

Figure 1.
Overview of the interactions between biochemical pathways common to pre-eclampsia and GDM.

statuses i.e. early- vs. late-onset pre-eclampsia and T1D, pre-existing T2DM, and GDM is required. To achieve this, prospective cohort studies need to be set up in which biochemical data is collected from women at pre-conception, at each trimester during pregnancy and post-partum (ideally with long-term follow-up). Gaining a better understanding of shared and separate pathophysiological pathways would help improve screening and treatment.

Conflict of interest

None.

Author details

Maria Portelli and Byron Baron*
Faculty of Medicine and Surgery, Centre for Molecular Medicine and Biobanking, University of Malta, Msida, Malta

*Address all correspondence to: byron.baron@um.edu.mt

References

[1] Portelli M, Baron B. Clinical presentation of preeclampsia and the diagnostic value of proteins and their methylation products as biomarkers in pregnant women with preeclampsia and their newborns. Journal of Pregnancy. 2018;**2018**:1-23

[2] Nelson DB, Ziadie MS, McIntire DD, Rogers BB, Leveno KJ. Placental pathology suggesting that preeclampsia is more than one disease. American Journal of Obstetrics and Gynecology. 2014;**210**(1):66-e1

[3] Jiwani A, Marseille E, Lohse N, Damm P, Hod M, Kahn JG. Gestational diabetes mellitus: Results from a survey of country prevalence and practices. The Journal of Maternal-Fetal and Neonatal Medicine. 2012;**25**(6):600-610

[4] Buchanan TA, Xiang AH. Gestational diabetes mellitus. The Journal of Clinical Investigation. 2005;**115**(3):485-491

[5] Schneider S, Freerksen N, Röhrig S, Hoeft B, Maul H. Gestational diabetes and preeclampsia–Similar risk factor profiles? Early Human Development. 2012;**88**(3):179-184

[6] Nerenberg KA, Johnson JA, Leung B, Savu A, Ryan EA, Chik CL, et al. Risks of gestational diabetes and preeclampsia over the last decade in a cohort of Alberta women. Journal of Obstetrics and Gynaecology Canada. 2013;**35**(11):986-994

[7] Lisonkova S, Joseph KS. Incidence of preeclampsia: Risk factors and outcomes associated with early-versus late-onset disease. American Journal of Obstetrics and Gynecology. 2013;**209**(6):544-5e1

[8] Weissgerber TL, Mudd LM. Preeclampsia and diabetes. Current Diabetes Reports. 2015;**15**(3):9

[9] Mudd LM, Owe KM, Mottola MF, Pivarnik JM. Health benefits of physical activity during pregnancy: An international perspective. Medicine and Science in Sports and Exercise. 2013;**45**(2):268-277

[10] Mastrogiannis DS, Spiliopoulos M, Mulla W, Homko CJ. Insulin resistance: The possible link between gestational diabetes mellitus and hypertensive disorders of pregnancy. Current Diabetes Reports. 2009;**9**(4):296

[11] Wen SW, Xie RH, Tan H, Walker MC, Smith GN, Retnakaran R. Preeclampsia and gestational diabetes mellitus: Pre-conception origins? Medical Hypotheses. 2012;**79**(1):120-125

[12] Roberts JM, Lain KY. Recent insights into the pathogenesis of pre-eclampsia. Placenta. 2002;**23**(5):359-372

[13] Jauniaux E, Hempstock J, Greenwold N, Burton GJ. Trophoblastic oxidative stress in relation to temporal and regional differences in maternal placental blood flow in normal and abnormal early pregnancies. The American Journal of Pathology. 2003;**162**(1):115-125

[14] Maynard SE, Min JY, Merchan J, Lim KH, Li J, Mondal S, et al. Excess placental soluble fms-like tyrosine kinase 1 (sFlt1) may contribute to endothelial dysfunction, hypertension, and proteinuria in preeclampsia. The Journal of Clinical Investigation. 2003;**111**(5):649-658

[15] Venkatesha S, Toporsian M, Lam C, Hanai JI, Mammoto T, Kim YM, et al. Soluble endoglin contributes to the pathogenesis of preeclampsia. Nature Medicine. 2006;**12**(6):642

[16] Mutter WP, Karumanchi SA. Molecular mechanisms of preeclampsia. Microvascular Research. 2008;**75**(1):1-8

[17] Chaiworapongsa T, Chaemsaithong P, Yeo L, Romero R. Pre-eclampsia part 1: Current understanding of its pathophysiology. Nature Reviews Nephrology. 2014;**10**(8):466

[18] Karumanchi SA. Angiogenic factors in preeclampsia: From diagnosis to therapy. Hypertension. 2016;**67**(6):1072-1079

[19] Levine RJ, Maynard SE, Qian C, Lim KH, England LJ, Kai FY, et al. Obstetric anesthesia. The New England Journal of Medicine. 2004;**350**:672-683

[20] Lai J, Larroca SG, Peeva G, Poon LC, Wright D, Nicolaides KH. Competing risks model in screening for preeclampsia by serum placental growth factor and soluble fms-like tyrosine kinase-1 at 30-33 weeks' gestation. Fetal Diagnosis and Therapy. 2014;**35**(4):240-248

[21] Tsiakkas A, Saiid Y, Wright A, Wright D, Nicolaides KH. Competing risks model in screening for preeclampsia by maternal factors and biomarkers at 30-34 weeks' gestation. American Journal of Obstetrics and Gynecology. 2016;**215**(1):87-e1

[22] Verlohren S, Stepan H, Dechend R. Angiogenic growth factors in the diagnosis and prediction of pre-eclampsia. Clinical Science. 2012;**122**(2):43-52

[23] Widmer M, Cuesta C, Khan KS, Conde-Agudelo A, Carroli G, Fusey S, et al. Accuracy of angiogenic biomarkers at 20 weeks' gestation in predicting the risk of pre-eclampsia: A WHO multicentre study. Pregnancy Hypertension: An International Journal of Women's Cardiovascular Health. 2015;**5**(4):330-338

[24] Khalil A, Maiz N, Garcia-Mandujano R, Penco JM, Nicolaides KH. Longitudinal changes in maternal serum placental growth factor and soluble fms-like tyrosine kinase-1 in women at increased risk of pre-eclampsia. Ultrasound in Obstetrics and Gynecology. 2016;**47**(3):324-331

[25] Chaiworapongsa T, Romero R, Whitten AE, Korzeniewski SJ, Chaemsaithong P, Hernandez-Andrade E, et al. The use of angiogenic biomarkers in maternal blood to identify which SGA fetuses will require a preterm delivery and mothers who will develop pre-eclampsia. The Journal of Maternal-Fetal and Neonatal Medicine. 2016;**29**(8):1214-1228

[26] Korzeniewski SJ, Romero R, Chaiworapongsa T, Chaemsaithong P, Kim CJ, Kim YM, et al. Maternal plasma angiogenic index-1 (placental growth factor/soluble vascular endothelial growth factor receptor-1) is a biomarker for the burden of placental lesions consistent with uteroplacental underperfusion: A longitudinal case-cohort study. American Journal of Obstetrics and Gynecology. 2016;**214**(5):629-6e1

[27] Zeisler H, Llurba E, Chantraine F, Vatish M, Staff AC, Sennström M, et al. Predictive value of the sFlt-1: PlGF ratio in women with suspected preeclampsia. New England Journal of Medicine. 2016;**374**(1):13-22

[28] Romero R, Erez O, Hüttemann M, Maymon E, Panaitescu B, Conde-Agudelo A, et al. Metformin, the aspirin of the 21st century: Its role in gestational diabetes mellitus, prevention of preeclampsia and cancer, and the promotion of longevity. American Journal of Obstetrics and Gynecology. 2017;**217**(3):282-302

[29] Portelli M. Measurement of asymmetric dimethyl-arginine (ADMA) and methyl-lysine levels in pregnant women with pre-eclampsia and their newborns [thesis]. Malta: University of Malta; 2018

[30] Powers RW, Jeyabalan A, Clifton RG, Van Dorsten P, Hauth JC, Klebanoff

MA, et al. Eunice Kennedy Shriver National Institute of Child Health Human Development Maternal-Fetal Medicine Units Network. Soluble fms-Like tyrosine kinase 1 (sFlt1), endoglin and placental growth factor (PlGF) in preeclampsia among high risk pregnancies. PloS One. 2010;**5**(10):e13263

[31] Rana S, Powe CE, Salahuddin S, Verlohren S, Perschel FH, Levine RJ, et al. Angiogenic factors and the risk of adverse outcomes in women with suspected preeclampsia. Circulation. 2012;**125**(7):911-919

[32] Baltajian K, Bajracharya S, Salahuddin S, Berg AH, Geahchan C, Wenger JB, et al. Sequential plasma angiogenic factors levels in women with suspected preeclampsia. American Journal of Obstetrics and Gynecology. 2016;**215**(1):89-e1

[33] Rana S, Karumanchi SA, Levine RJ, Venkatesha S, Rauh-Hain JA, Tamez H, et al. Sequential changes in antiangiogenic factors in early pregnancy and risk of developing preeclampsia. Hypertension. 2007;**50**(1):137-142

[34] Zhao B, Han X, Meng Q, Luo Q. Early second trimester maternal serum markers in the prediction of gestational diabetes mellitus. Journal of Diabetes Investigation. 2018;**9**(4):967-974

[35] Sun X, Qu T, He X, Yang X, Guo N, Mao Y, et al. Screening of differentially expressed proteins from syncytiotrophoblast for severe early-onset preeclampsia in women with gestational diabetes mellitus using tandem mass tag quantitative proteomics. BMC Pregnancy and Childbirth. 2018;**18**(1):437

[36] Bonney EA. Preeclampsia: A view through the danger model. Journal of Reproductive Immunology. 2007;**76**(1-2):68-74

[37] Kim YM, Romero R, Oh SY, Kim CJ, Kilburn BA, Armant DR, et al. Toll-like receptor 4: A potential link between "danger signals," the innate immune system, and preeclampsia? American Journal of Obstetrics and Gynecology. 2005;**193**(3):921-9e1

[38] Barbour LA, McCurdy CE, Hernandez TL, Kirwan JP, Catalano PM, Friedman JE. Cellular mechanisms for insulin resistance in normal pregnancy and gestational diabetes. Diabetes Care. 2007;**30**(Supplement 2):S112-S119

[39] Villalobos-Labra R, Silva L, Subiabre M, Araos J, Salsoso R, Fuenzalida B, et al. Akt/mTOR role in human foetoplacental vascular insulin resistance in diseases of pregnancy. Journal of Diabetes Research. 2017;**2017**:1-13

[40] Valdés E, Sepúlveda-Martínez Á, Manukián B, Parra-Cordero M. Assessment of pregestational insulin resistance as a risk factor of preeclampsia. Gynecologic and Obstetric Investigation. 2014;**77**(2):111-116

[41] Hauth JC, Clifton RG, Roberts JM, Myatt L, Spong CY, Leveno KJ, et al. Maternal insulin resistance and preeclampsia. Obstetric Anesthesia Digest. 2012;**32**(1):42-43

[42] Alsnes IV, Janszky I, Forman MR, Vatten LJ, Økland I. A population-based study of associations between preeclampsia and later cardiovascular risk factors. American Journal of Obstetrics and Gynecology. 2014;**211**(6):657-6e1

[43] Gunderson EP, Quesenberry CP Jr, Jacobs DR Jr, Feng J, Lewis CE, Sidney S. Longitudinal study of prepregnancy cardiometabolic risk factors and subsequent risk of gestational diabetes mellitus: The CARDIA study. American Journal of Epidemiology. 2010;**172**(10):1131-1143

[44] Reece EA, Leguizamón G, Wiznitzer A. Gestational diabetes: The need for a common ground. The Lancet. 2009;**373**(9677):1789-1797

[45] Yang X, Guo L, Li H, Chen X, Tong X. Analysis of the original causes of placental oxidative stress in normal pregnancy and pre-eclampsia: A hypothesis. The Journal of Maternal-Fetal and Neonatal Medicine. 2012;**25**(7):884-888

[46] Karacay Ö, Sepici-Dincel A, Karcaaltincaba D, Sahin D, Yalvaç S, Akyol M, et al. A quantitative evaluation of total antioxidant status and oxidative stress markers in preeclampsia and gestational diabetic patients in 24-36 weeks of gestation. Diabetes Research and Clinical Practice. 2010;**89**(3):231-238

[47] Burton GJ, Jauniaux E. Oxidative stress. Best Practice and Research Clinical Obstetrics and Gynaecology. 2011;**25**(3):287-299

[48] Lappas M, Hiden U, Desoye G, Froehlich J, Mouzon SH, Jawerbaum A. The role of oxidative stress in the pathophysiology of gestational diabetes mellitus. Antioxidants and Redox Signaling. 2011;**15**(12):3061-3100

[49] Bilodeau JF. Maternal and placental antioxidant response to preeclampsia–impact on vasoactive eicosanoids. Placenta. 2014;**35**:S32-S38

[50] Sánchez-Aranguren LC, Prada CE, Riaño-Medina CE, Lopez M. Endothelial dysfunction and preeclampsia: Role of oxidative stress. Frontiers in Physiology. 2014;**5**:372

[51] Khaing W, Vallibhakara SA, Tantrakul V, Vallibhakara O, Rattanasiri S, McEvoy M, et al. Calcium and vitamin D supplementation for prevention of preeclampsia: A systematic review and network meta-analysis. Nutrients. 2017;**9**(10):1141

[52] Giacco F, Brownlee M. Oxidative stress and diabetic complications. Circulation Research. 2010;**107**(9):1058-1070

[53] Rao R, Sen S, Han B, Ramadoss S, Chaudhuri G. Gestational diabetes, preeclampsia and cytokine release: Similarities and Differences in Endothelial Cell Function. In: Advances in Fetal and Neonatal Physiology. New York, NY: Springer; 2014. pp. 69-75

[54] Rashid G, Benchetrit S, Fishman D, Bernheim J. Effect of advanced glycation end-products on gene expression and synthesis of TNF-α and endothelial nitric oxide synthase by endothelial cells. Kidney International. 2004;**66**(3):1099-1106

[55] Xu B, Ji Y, Yao K, Cao YX, Ferro A. Inhibition of human endothelial cell nitric oxide synthesis by advanced glycation end-products but not glucose: Relevance to diabetes. Clinical Science. 2005;**109**(5):439-446

[56] Yan JY, Jiang LL. Expression of advanced glycation end products in placenta and concentration in maternal and umbilical serum in pre-eclampsia. Journal of Obstetrics and Gynaecology Research. 2015;**41**(6):843-849

[57] Xian N, Chen W, Zhang Y, Li J, Zhang N, Ye Y. Correlation of the expressions of advanced glycation end products and its receptor in serum and placenta with the pathogenesis of preeclampsia. Zhonghua Fu Chan Ke Za Zhi. 2015;**50**(7):493-499

[58] Chen W, Zhang Y, Yue C, Ye Y, Chen P, Peng W, et al. Accumulation of advanced glycation end products involved in inflammation and contributing to severe preeclampsia, in maternal blood, umbilical blood and placental tissues. Gynecologic and Obstetric Investigation. 2017;**82**(4):388-397

[59] Huang QT, Zhang M, Zhong M, Yu YH, Liang WZ, Hang LL, et al. Advanced glycation end products as an upstream molecule triggers ROS-induced sFlt-1 production in extravillous trophoblasts: A novel bridge between oxidative stress and preeclampsia. Placenta. 2013;**34**(12):1177-1182

[60] Genc H, Uzun H, Benian A, Simsek G, Gelisgen R, Madazli R, et al. Evaluation of oxidative stress markers in first trimester for assessment of preeclampsia risk. Archives of Gynecology and Obstetrics. 2011;**284**(6):1367-1373

[61] Arribas L, Almansa I, Miranda M, Muriach M, Romero FJ, Villar VM. Serum malondialdehyde concentration and glutathione peroxidase activity in a longitudinal study of gestational diabetes. PLoS One. 2016;**11**(5):e0155353

[62] Vishnyakova PA, Volodina MA, Tarasova NV, Marey MV, Tsvirkun DV, Vavina OV, et al. Mitochondrial role in adaptive response to stress conditions in preeclampsia. Scientific Reports. 2016;**6**:32410

[63] Shi Z, Long W, Zhao C, Guo X, Shen R, Ding H. Comparative proteomics analysis suggests that placental mitochondria are involved in the development of pre-eclampsia. PLoS One. 2013;**8**(5):e64351

[64] Mihu D, Razvan C, Malutan A, Mihaela C. Evaluation of maternal systemic inflammatory response in preeclampsia. Taiwanese Journal of Obstetrics and Gynecology. 2015;**54**(2):160-166

[65] Weel IC, Baergen RN, Romão-Veiga M, Borges VT, Ribeiro VR, Witkin SS, et al. Association between placental lesions, cytokines and angiogenic factors in pregnant women with preeclampsia. PLoS One. 2016;**11**(6):e0157584

[66] Wolf M, Sauk J, Shah A, Smirnakis KV, Jimenez-Kimble R, Ecker JL, et al. Inflammation and glucose intolerance: A prospective study of gestational diabetes mellitus. Diabetes Care. 2004;**27**(1):21-27

[67] Kirwan JP, Hauguel-De Mouzon S, Lepercq J, Challier JC, Huston-Presley L, Friedman JE, et al. TNF-α is a predictor of insulin resistance in human pregnancy. Diabetes. 2002;**51**(7):2207-2213

[68] McLachlan KA, O'neal D, Jenkins A, Alford FP. Do adiponectin, TNFα, leptin and CRP relate to insulin resistance in pregnancy? Studies in women with and without gestational diabetes, during and after pregnancy. Diabetes/Metabolism Research and Reviews. 2006;**22**(2):131-138

[69] Atègbo JM, Grissa O, Yessoufou A, Hichami A, Dramane KL, Moutairou K, et al. Modulation of adipokines and cytokines in gestational diabetes and macrosomia. The Journal of Clinical Endocrinology and Metabolism. 2006;**91**(10):4137-4143

[70] Heitritter SM, Solomon CG, Mitchell GF, Skali-Ounis N, Seely EW. Subclinical inflammation and vascular dysfunction in women with previous gestational diabetes mellitus. The Journal of Clinical Endocrinology and Metabolism. 2005;**90**(7):3983-3988

[71] Miehle K, Stepan H, Fasshauer M. Leptin, adiponectin and other adipokines in gestational diabetes mellitus and pre-eclampsia. Clinical Endocrinology. 2012;**76**(1):2-11

[72] Phaloprakarn C, Tangjitgamol S. Risk assessment for preeclampsia in women with gestational diabetes mellitus. Journal of Perinatal Medicine. 2009;**37**(6):617-621

[73] Knight KM, Pressman EK, Hackney DN, Thornburg LL. Perinatal outcomes

in type 2 diabetic patients compared with non-diabetic patients matched by body mass index. The Journal of Maternal-Fetal and Neonatal Medicine. 2012;**25**(6):611-615

[74] Jeyabalan A. Epidemiology of preeclampsia: Impact of obesity. Nutrition Reviews. 2013;**71**(suppl_1):S18-S25

[75] Zavalza-Gómez AB, Anaya-Prado R, Rincón-Sánchez AR, Mora-Martínez JM. Adipokines and insulin resistance during pregnancy. Diabetes Research and Clinical Practice. 2008;**80**(1):8-15

[76] Ahima RS, Flier JS. Leptin. Annual Review of Physiology. 2000;**62**(1):413-437

[77] Hendler I, Blackwell SC, Mehta SH, Whitty JE, Russell E, Sorokin Y, et al. The levels of leptin, adiponectin, and resistin in normal weight, overweight, and obese pregnant women with and without preeclampsia. American Journal of Obstetrics and Gynecology. 2005;**193**(3):979-983

[78] Ramsay JE, Jamieson N, Greer IA, Sattar N. Paradoxical elevation in adiponectin concentrations in women with preeclampsia. Hypertension. 2003;**42**(5):891-894

[79] Kajantie E, Kaaja R, Ylikorkala O, Andersson S, Laivouri H. Adiponectin concentrations in maternal serum: Elevated in preeclampsis but unrelated to insulin sensitivity. Journal of the Society for Gynecologic Investigation. 2005;**12**(6):433-439

[80] Naruse K, Yamasaki M, Umekage H, Sado T, Sakamoto Y, Morikawa H. Peripheral blood concentrations of adiponectin, an adipocyte-specific plasma protein, in normal pregnancy and preeclampsia. Journal of Reproductive Immunology. 2005;**65**(1):65-75

[81] Fazeli Daryasari SR, Razavinia F, Tork Tatari F, Pahlevan F, Tehranian N. The role of adiponectin in gestational diabetes mellitus, preeclampsia and obesity during pregnancy: A systematic review. Iranian Journal of Endocrinology and Metabolism. 2018;**19**(5):370-383

[82] Chen J, Tan B, Karteris E, Zervou S, Digby J, Hillhouse EW, et al. Secretion of adiponectin by human placenta: Differential modulation of adiponectin and its receptors by cytokines. Diabetologia. 2006;**49**(6):1292

[83] Altinova AE, Toruner F, Bozkurt N, Bukan N, Karakoc A, Yetkin I, et al. Circulating concentrations of adiponectin and tumor necrosis factor-α in gestational diabetes mellitus. Gynecological Endocrinology. 2007;**23**(3):161-165

[84] Retnakaran R, Connelly PW, Maguire G, Sermer M, Zinman B, Hanley AJ. Decreased high-molecular-weight adiponectin in gestational diabetes: Implications for the pathophysiology of Type 2 diabetes. Diabetic Medicine. 2007;**24**(3):245-252

[85] Thagaard IN, Krebs L, Holm JC, Lange T, Larsen T, Christiansen M. Adiponectin and leptin as first trimester markers for gestational diabetes mellitus: A cohort study. Clinical Chemistry and Laboratory Medicine (CCLM). 2017;**55**(11):1805-1812

[86] Retnakaran R, Qi Y, Connelly PW, Sermer M, Hanley AJ, Zinman B. Low adiponectin concentration during pregnancy predicts postpartum insulin resistance, beta cell dysfunction and fasting glycaemia. Diabetologia. 2010;**53**(2):268

[87] Haugen F, Ranheim T, Harsem NK, Lips E, Staff AC, Drevon CA. Increased plasma levels of adipokines in preeclampsia: Relationship to placenta and adipose tissue gene expression.

American Journal of Physiology-Endocrinology and Metabolism. 2006;**290**(2):E326-333

[88] Adali E, Yildizhan R, Kolusari A, Kurdoglu M, Bugdayci G, Sahin HG, et al. Increased visfatin and leptin in pregnancies complicated by pre-eclampsia. The Journal of Maternal-Fetal and Neonatal Medicine. 2009;**22**(10):873-879

[89] Masuyama H, Segawa T, Sumida Y, Masumoto A, Inoue S, Akahori Y, et al. Different profiles of circulating angiogenic factors and adipocytokines between early-and late-onset pre-eclampsia. BJOG: An International Journal of Obstetrics and Gynaecology. 2010;**117**(3):314-320

[90] Anim-Nyame N, Sooranna SR, Steer PJ, Johnson MR. Longitudinal analysis of maternal plasma leptin concentrations during normal pregnancy and pre-eclampsia. Human Reproduction. 2000;**15**(9):2033-2036

[91] Chappell LC, Seed PT, Briley A, Kelly FJ, Hunt BJ, Charnock-Jones DS, et al. A longitudinal study of biochemical variables in women at risk of preeclampsia. American Journal of Obstetrics and Gynecology. 2002;**187**(1):127-136

[92] Ning Y, Williams MA, Muy-Rivera M, Leisenring WM, Luthy DA. Relationship of maternal plasma leptin and risk of pre-eclampsia: A prospective study. The Journal of Maternal-Fetal and Neonatal Medicine. 2004;**15**(3):186-192

[93] Samolis S, Papastefanou I, Panagopoulos P, Galazios G, Kouskoukis A, Maroulis G. Relation between first trimester maternal serum leptin levels and body mass index in normotensive and pre-eclamptic pregnancies–role of leptin as a marker of pre-eclampsia: A prospective case–control study. Gynecological Endocrinology. 2010;**26**(5):338-343

[94] Kautzky-Willer A, Pacini G, Tura A, Bieglmayer C, Schneider B, Ludvik B, et al. Increased plasma leptin in gestational diabetes. Diabetologia. 2001;**44**(2):164-172

[95] Vitoratos N, Salamalekis E, Kassanos D, Loghis C, Panayotopoulos N, Kouskouni E, et al. Maternal plasma leptin levels and their relationship to insulin and glucose in gestational-onset diabetes. Gynecologic and Obstetric Investigation. 2001;**51**(1):17-21

[96] Chen D, Xia G, Xu P, Dong M. Peripartum serum leptin and soluble leptin receptor levels in women with gestational diabetes. Acta Obstetricia et Gynecologica Scandinavica. 2010;**89**(12):1595-1599

[97] Hauguel-de Mouzon S, Lepercq J, Catalano P. The known and unknown of leptin in pregnancy. American Journal of Obstetrics and Gynecology. 2006;**194**(6):1537-1545

[98] Ouchi N, Parker JL, Lugus JJ, Walsh K. Adipokines in inflammation and metabolic disease. Nature Reviews Immunology. 2011;**11**(2):85

[99] Jawerbaum A, Capobianco E. Effects of PPAR activation in the placenta and the fetus: Implications in maternal diabetes. Placenta. 2011;**32**:S212-S217

[100] Waite LL, Person EC, Zhou Y, Lim KH, Scanlan TS, Taylor RN. Placental peroxisome proliferator-activated receptor-γ is up-regulated by pregnancy serum. The Journal of Clinical Endocrinology and Metabolism. 2000;**85**(10):3808-3814

[101] Waite LL, Louie RE, Taylor RN. Circulating activators of peroxisome proliferator-activated receptors are reduced in preeclamptic pregnancy. The Journal of Clinical Endocrinology and Metabolism. 2005;**90**(2):620-626

[102] McCarthy FP, Drewlo S, English FA, Kingdom J, Johns EJ, Kenny LC, et al. Evidence implicating peroxisome proliferator-activated receptor-γ in the pathogenesis of preeclampsia. Hypertension. 2011;**58**(5):882-887

[103] McCarthy FP, Drewlo S, Kingdom J, Johns EJ, Walsh SK, Kenny LC. Peroxisome proliferator-activated receptor-γ as a potential therapeutic target in the treatment of preeclampsia. Hypertension. 2011;**58**(2):280-286

[104] Holdsworth-Carson SJ, Lim R, Mitton A, Whitehead C, Rice GE, Permezel M, et al. Peroxisome proliferator-activated receptors are altered in pathologies of the human placenta: Gestational diabetes mellitus, intrauterine growth restriction and preeclampsia. Placenta. 2010;**31**(3):222-229

[105] Salzer L, Tenenbaum-Gavish K, Hod M. Metabolic disorder of pregnancy (understanding pathophysiology of diabetes and preeclampsia). Best Practice and Research Clinical Obstetrics and Gynaecology. 2015;**29**(3):328-338

[106] Leavey K, Benton SJ, Grynspan D, Kingdom JC, Bainbridge SA, Cox BJ. Unsupervised placental gene expression profiling identifies clinically relevant subclasses of human preeclampsia. Hypertension. 2016;**68**(1):137-147

[107] Lowe WL, Scholtens DM, Sandler V, Hayes MG. Genetics of gestational diabetes mellitus and maternal metabolism. Current Diabetes Reports. 2016;**16**(2):15

[108] Wu L, Cui L, Tam WH, Ma RC, Wang CC. Genetic variants associated with gestational diabetes mellitus: A meta-analysis and subgroup analysis. Scientific Reports. 2016;**6**:30539

[109] Enquobahrie DA, Williams MA, Qiu C, Meller M, Sorensen TK. Global placental gene expression in gestational diabetes mellitus. American Journal of Obstetrics and Gynecology. 2009;**200**(2):206-2e1

[110] Cutfield WS, Hofman PL, Mitchell M, Morison IM. Could epigenetics play a role in the developmental origins of health and disease? Pediatric Research. 2007;**61**(5 Part 2):68R

[111] Schroeder DI, Jayashankar K, Douglas KC, Thirkill TL, York D, Dickinson PJ, et al. Early developmental and evolutionary origins of gene body DNA methylation patterns in mammalian placentas. PLoS Genetics. 2015;**11**(8):e1005442

[112] Jia RZ, Zhang X, Hu P, Liu XM, Hua XD, Wang X, et al. Screening for differential methylation status in human placenta in preeclampsia using a CpG island plus promoter microarray. International Journal of Molecular Medicine. 2012;**30**(1):133-141

[113] Ruchat SM, Houde AA, Voisin G, St-Pierre J, Perron P, Baillargeon JP, et al. Gestational diabetes mellitus epigenetically affects genes predominantly involved in metabolic diseases. Epigenetics. 2013;**8**(9):935-943

[114] Blair JD, Yuen RK, Lim BK, McFadden DE, von Dadelszen P, Robinson WP. Widespread DNA hypomethylation at gene enhancer regions in placentas associated with early-onset pre-eclampsia. Molecular Human Reproduction. 2013;**19**(10):697-708

[115] Anton L, Brown AG, Bartolomei MS, Elovitz MA. Differential methylation of genes associated with cell adhesion in preeclamptic placentas. PLoS One. 2014;**9**(6):e100148

[116] Chu T, Bunce K, Shaw P, Shridhar V, Althouse A, Hubel

C, et al. Comprehensive analysis of preeclampsia-associated DNA methylation in the placenta. PLoS One. 2014;**9**(9):e107318

[117] Liu L, Zhang X, Rong C, Rui C, Ji H, Qian YJ, et al. Distinct DNA methylomes of human placentas between pre-eclampsia and gestational diabetes mellitus. Cellular Physiology and Biochemistry. 2014;**34**(6):1877-1889

[118] Petropoulos S, Guillemin C, Ergaz Z, Dimov S, Suderman M, Weinstein-Fudim L, et al. Gestational diabetes alters offspring DNA methylation profiles in human and rat: Identification of key pathways involved in endocrine system disorders, insulin signaling, diabetes signaling, and ILK signaling. Endocrinology. 2015;**156**(6):2222-2238

[119] Finer S, Mathews C, Lowe R, Smart M, Hillman S, Foo L, et al. Maternal gestational diabetes is associated with genome-wide DNA methylation variation in placenta and cord blood of exposed offspring. Human Molecular Genetics. 2015;**24**(11):3021-3029

[120] Binder AM, LaRocca J, Lesseur C, Marsit CJ, Michels KB. Epigenome-wide and transcriptome-wide analyses reveal gestational diabetes is associated with alterations in the human leukocyte antigen complex. Clinical Epigenetics. 2015;**7**(1):79

[121] Nomura Y, Lambertini L, Rialdi A, Lee M, Mystal EY, Grabie M, et al. Global methylation in the placenta and umbilical cord blood from pregnancies with maternal gestational diabetes, preeclampsia, and obesity. Reproductive Sciences. 2014;**21**(1):131-137

[122] Reichetzeder C, Putra SD, Pfab T, Slowinski T, Neuber C, Kleuser B, et al. Increased global placental DNA methylation levels are associated with gestational diabetes. Clinical Epigenetics. 2016;**8**(1):82

[123] Williams KT, Schalinske KL. Tissue-specific alterations of methyl group metabolism with DNA hypermethylation in the Zucker (type 2) diabetic fatty rat. Diabetes/Metabolism Research and Reviews. 2012;**28**(2):123-131

[124] Rani V, Deep G, Singh RK, Palle K, Yadav UC. Oxidative stress and metabolic disorders: Pathogenesis and therapeutic strategies. Life Sciences. 2016;**148**:183-193

[125] Zhong J, Xu C, Reece EA, Yang P. The green tea polyphenol EGCG alleviates maternal diabetes–induced neural tube defects by inhibiting DNA hypermethylation. American Journal of Obstetrics and Gynecology. 2016;**215**(3):368-3e1

[126] Morales-Prieto DM, Chaiwangyen W, Ospina-Prieto S, Schneider U, Herrmann J, Gruhn B, et al. MicroRNA expression profiles of trophoblastic cells. Placenta. 2012;**33**(9):725-734

[127] Chim SS, Shing TK, Hung EC, Leung TY, Lau TK, Chiu RW, et al. Detection and characterization of placental microRNAs in maternal plasma. Clinical Chemistry. 2008;**54**(3):482-490

[128] Li H, Ge Q, Guo L, Lu Z. Maternal plasma miRNAs expression in preeclamptic pregnancies. BioMed Research International. 2013;**2013**:1-9

[129] Pineles BL, Romero R, Montenegro D, Tarca AL, Han YM, Kim YM, et al. Distinct subsets of microRNAs are expressed differentially in the human placentas of patients with preeclampsia. American Journal of Obstetrics and Gynecology. 2007;**196**(3):261-2e1

[130] Zhu XM, Han T, Sargent IL, Yin GW, Yao YQ. Differential expression profile of microRNAs in human placentas from preeclamptic pregnancies vs normal pregnancies.

American Journal of Obstetrics and Gynecology. 2009;**200**(6):661-6e1

[131] Hu Y, Li P, Hao S, Liu L, Zhao J, Hou Y. Differential expression of microRNAs in the placentae of Chinese patients with severe pre-eclampsia. Clinical Chemistry and Laboratory Medicine. 2009;**47**(8):923-929

[132] Enquobahrie DA, Abetew DF, Sorensen TK, Willoughby D, Chidambaram K, Williams MA. Placental microRNA expression in pregnancies complicated by preeclampsia. American Journal of Obstetrics and Gynecology. 2011;**204**(2):178-e12

[133] Muralimanoharan S, Maloyan A, Mele J, Guo C, Myatt LG, Myatt L. MIR-210 modulates mitochondrial respiration in placenta with preeclampsia. Placenta. 2012;**33**(10):816-823

[134] Betoni JS, Derr K, Pahl MC, Rogers L, Muller CL, Packard RE, et al. MicroRNA analysis in placentas from patients with preeclampsia: Comparison of new and published results. Hypertension in Pregnancy. 2013;**32**(4):321-339

[135] Zhang Y, Fei M, Xue G, Zhou Q, Jia Y, Li L, et al. Elevated levels of hypoxia-inducible microRNA-210 in pre-eclampsia: New insights into molecular mechanisms for the disease. Journal of Cellular and Molecular Medicine. 2012;**16**(2):249-259

[136] Zhao C, Dong J, Jiang T, Shi Z, Yu B, Zhu Y, et al. Early second-trimester serum miRNA profiling predicts gestational diabetes mellitus. PLoS One. 2011;**6**(8):e23925

[137] Zhu Y, Tian F, Li H, Zhou Y, Lu J, Ge Q. Profiling maternal plasma microRNA expression in early pregnancy to predict gestational diabetes mellitus. International Journal of Gynecology and Obstetrics. 2015;**130**(1):49-53

[138] Li J, Song L, Zhou L, Wu J, Sheng C, Chen H, et al. A microRNA signature in gestational diabetes mellitus associated with risk of macrosomia. Cellular Physiology and Biochemistry. 2015;**37**(1):243-252

[139] Tryggestad JB, Vishwanath A, Jiang S, Mallappa A, Teague AM, Takahashi Y, et al. Influence of gestational diabetes mellitus on human umbilical vein endothelial cell miRNA. Clinical Science. 2016;**130**(21):1955-1967

[140] Collares CV, Evangelista AF, Xavier DJ, Rassi DM, Arns T, Foss-Freitas MC, et al. Identifying common and specific microRNAs expressed in peripheral blood mononuclear cell of type 1, type 2, and gestational diabetes mellitus patients. BMC Research Notes. 2013;**6**(1):491

[141] Floris I, Descamps B, Vardeu A, Mitić T, Posadino AM, Shantikumar S, et al. Gestational diabetes mellitus impairs fetal endothelial cell functions through a mechanism involving microRNA-101 and histone methyltransferase enhancer of zester homolog-2. Arteriosclerosis, Thrombosis, and Vascular Biology. 2015;**35**(3):664-674

[142] Nanovskaya TN, Nekhayeva IA, Patrikeeva SL, Hankins GD, Ahmed MS. Transfer of metformin across the dually perfused human placental lobule. American Journal of Obstetrics and Gynecology. 2006;**195**(4):1081-1085

[143] Cassina M, Dona M, Di Gianantonio E, Litta P, Clementi M. First-trimester exposure to metformin and risk of birth defects: A systematic review and meta-analysis. Human Reproduction Update. 2014;**20**(5):656-669

[144] Foretz M, Guigas B, Bertrand L, Pollak M, Viollet B. Metformin: From

mechanisms of action to therapies. Cell Metabolism. 2014;**20**(6):953-966

[145] Ainuddin J, Karim N, Hasan AA, Naqvi SA. Metformin versus insulin treatment in gestational diabetes in pregnancy in a developing country. A randomized control trial. Diabetes Research and Clinical Practice. 2015;**107**(2):290-299

[146] Butalia S, Gutierrez L, Lodha A, Aitken E, Zakariasen A, Donovan L. Short-and long-term outcomes of metformin compared with insulin alone in pregnancy: A systematic review and meta-analysis. Diabetic Medicine. 2017;**34**(1):27-36

[147] Alqudah A, McKinley MC, McNally R, Graham U, Watson CJ, Lyons TJ, et al. Risk of pre-eclampsia in women taking metformin: A systematic review and meta-analysis. Diabetic Medicine. 2018;**35**(2):160-172

[148] Brownfoot FC, Hastie R, Hannan NJ, Cannon P, Tuohey L, Parry LJ, et al. Metformin as a prevention and treatment for preeclampsia: Effects on soluble fms-like tyrosine kinase 1 and soluble endoglin secretion and endothelial dysfunction. American Journal of Obstetrics and Gynecology. 2016;**214**(3):356-3e1

Chapter 8

Adolescence and Preeclampsia

Sergio Rosales-Ortiz, Olivia Sánchez Rodríguez, Mario Borbolla-Ramos and Karen D. García-Pérez

Abstract

Adolescent pregnancy is defined as that which occurs in a woman between 10 and 19 years of age. Approximately 10% of all women aged 15–19 become pregnant. It is estimated that 11% of births worldwide occur in this population. In teenage population, preeclampsia has a prevalence twice as high as that in adult population. Adolescent population is exposed to different maternal-fetal adverse outcomes such as preterm birth, low birth weight, and gestational diabetes mellitus, associated with the outcomes of preeclampsia like seizures, pulmonary edema, defects in coagulation, liver or kidney failure, and death. The risk of adverse outcome remained increased in adolescent compared to young adult mothers (20–24 years). That is why it's important to know the approach of preeclampsia in adolescent pregnancy. We will describe the principal chance in the adolescent pregnancy, related risk factors, major complications for mother and fetus, and management and late complication for both.

Keywords: adolescent pregnancy, preeclampsia

1. Introduction

Pregnancy at any age constitutes a very important biopsychosocial event, but in adolescence it encompasses a series of situations that may place the mother's and the fetus' health at risk, thus becoming a public health issue not only in the present but also in the future due to potential complications and as a reflection of the social conditions of a country.

Maternal, late fetal, neonatal, and infant mortalities have the highest rates in women under 20 years of age than in any other reproductive period.

Complications in adolescent mothers are a constant dilemma since many factors are involved, such as inadequate prenatal control, race, family factors, and economic and sociodemographic conditions.

Hypertensive problems associated with pregnancy are another public health issue that in developing countries still represent the first cause of maternal death; worldwide, their prevalence varies but hovers around 10% of all pregnancies.

Whatever causes triggering complications, maternal and neonatal deaths are significant indicators in all countries, and in the case of pregnant adolescents, developing preeclampsia and their high and varied worldwide prevalence make this combination, specifically this group of patients, a point of reference when establishing health policies.

IntechOpen

2. Definition of adolescence

The WHO defines adolescence as the period of human growth and development after childhood and before adulthood, between the ages of 10 and 19. It is one of the most important transitional phases in human life, characterized by an accelerated rhythm of growth and changes, only surpassed by those in infants. This growth and development phase is conditioned by several biological processes. The beginning of puberty is the hallmark of passage from childhood to adolescence. From this stage on, the reproductive system's capacity to procreate is potentially latent [1].

3. Classification of adolescence

It is difficult to establish the chronological boundaries of this period, but in accordance with conventionally accepted concepts accepted by the World Health Organization (WHO), adolescence may be divided into two phases:

1. Early (10–14 years).

2. Late (15–19 years).

Likewise, other authors refer that there are three stages:

1. Early adolescence, between the ages of 10 and 13.

2. Mid-adolescence, between the ages of 14 and 17.

3. Late adolescence, between the ages of 17 and 21 [2].

4. Impact of pregnancy on an adolescent

The beginning of sexual activity in adolescents currently occurs at a younger age and carries immediate unwanted consequences such as an increased frequency of sexually transmitted diseases (STD) and unwanted pregnancy that may lead to miscarriage or other complications during pregnancy [3].

From a biological viewpoint, some of the consequences of adolescent pregnancy include hypertensive disease of pregnancy, anemia, gestational diabetes, and complications during childbirth that lead to an increase in maternal and fetal mortality [4]; complications in the newborn include higher rates of low birth weight, premature delivery, respiratory diseases, dystocia, and an increased frequency of neonatal complications and greater infant mortality [5].

Risk factors in adolescent pregnancy include low educational level, beginning sexual activity before the age of 15, absence of the partner, maternal history of pregnancy in adolescence, and the lack of knowledge and access to birth control methods. There is also a high percentage of school dropouts, a lack of plans for the future, low self-esteem, alcohol and drug abuse, ignorance on sexuality, and an inadequate use of birth control [6].

A correlation has been shown between minimal or absent family communication on birth control and sexuality and a higher risk of adolescent pregnancy and infection with sexually transmitted diseases [7].

Medical risks associated with pregnancy in adolescent mothers such as hypertensive pathology, anemia, low birth weight, prematurity, insufficient nutrition, etc. lead to an increase in maternal morbidity and mortality and an estimated two- to threefold increase in infant mortality among patients in the age range between 20 and 29.

In adolescents, the higher observed compared risk does not appear to be due to special physiologic conditions but to sociocultural variables and the medical care provided to these patients.

These pregnancies are frequently unwanted or unplanned events within a weak couple relationship, which leads to an attitude of rejection and concealment because of fear of the family group that, in turn, conditions late or insufficient prenatal care.

According to various publications, we must emphasize that 73–93% of cases of pregnant adolescents are women bearing their first child. The first pregnancy carries specific risks resulting from physiological immaturity in the pregnant

		<16 years		**>16 years**	
Kawakita [37]	CS	OR = 0.49; CI 95% = 0.42–0.59		OR = 0.75; CI 95% = 0.71–0.79	
	CA	OR = 0.63; CI 95% = 0.47–0.84		OR = 0.83; CI 95% = 0.75–0.91	
	MA	OR = 1.25; CI 95% = 1.07–1.45		OR = 1.15; CI 95% = 1.09–1.22	
	PD < 37 weeks	OR = 1.36; CI 95% = 1.14–1.62		aOR = 1.16; CI 95% = 1.08–1.25	
	PPH* and BT**	*OR = 1.46; CI 95% = 1.10–1.95		**OR = 1.21; CI 95% = 1.02–1.43	
	Preeclampsia and HELLP Sd	OR = 1.44; CI 95% = 1.17–1.77			
	PL			OR = 0.82; CI 95% = 0.71–0.95	
Bostanci et al. [21]		Early adolescent (%)	Late adolescent (%)	Adult (%)	P value
	Preeclampsia	4.8	2.7	5.9	<0.001
	PD	37.2	12.8	2.2	<0.001
	PPROM	37.2	10.2	8.5	<0.001
	IUGR	9	3.3	5.4	<0.001
	Postterm	0.7	5.9	8.7	<0.001
	Episiotomy	79.3	69.8	70	>0.05
	NICU	18	11.7	10	0.009
	Neonatal outcome	2.1	1.1	2.1	>0.05
	LBW	17.9	13.2	13.1	>0.05
	VLBW	4.1	3.4	2.7	>0.05
	CS	17.2	25.7	29.6	0.001

CS, cesarean section; CA, chorioamnionitis; MA, maternal anemia; PD, preterm delivery; PPH, postpartum hemorrhage; BT, blood transfusion; PL, perineal laceration; PPROM, preterm premature rupture of membranes; IUGR, intrauterine growth restriction; NICU, neonatal intensive care unit admission; LBW, low birth weight; VLBW, very low birth weight.

Table 1.
Comparison of some pregnancy complications and outcome among early and late adolescent.

adolescent. For example, preeclampsia or gestation-induced hypertension is more frequent in young pregnant women, from a low socioeconomic level, and specifically, in the first pregnancy, conditions all frequently met by a pregnant adolescent. When developing this clinical entity, a possible failure in the adaptive immune response has been posited, although it normally permits the development of a close interrelation between the maternal organism and its host. Since 50% of the fetal antigenic structure is of paternal origin, it acts like a graft and has been associated to factors such as immaturity of the maternal immune system or a functional abnormality that may be associated to maternal malnutrition, a very common condition in pregnant adolescents. Morbidity may be classified according to the gestational periods, whereby miscarriage, anemia, urinary tract infections, and asymptomatic bacteriuria are more common in the first half. In the second half, there are hypertensive manifestations, hemorrhage associated to placental pathology, scarce weight gain and associated maternal malnutrition, symptoms of premature delivery (abnormal contractility), and premature membrane rupture [8, 9].

Several authors have suggested that there is a relation between hypertensive disorders and pregnancy, which will be further discussed in this chapter. Other complications are summarized in **Table 1**.

A strategy to confront these problems and adolescent pregnancy is to increase the availability of high-quality sexual and reproductive health services for adolescents [10].

5. Frequency of preeclampsia in adolescents

Preeclampsia refers to a relatively common hypertensive disorder during pregnancy that develops progressively. Its cause remains unknown, and it frequently leads to severe maternal and perinatal complications.

Its incidence is broad since it depends on various aspects such as geographic location, race, nutritional or immunological factors, and associated comorbidities, and even a humid and cold climate has been related to a higher incidence of affected women.

It is estimated that about 7% of pregnancies will develop preeclampsia. The incidence of preeclampsia is about 25% in primiparous women. In industrialized nations, the rate of maternal morbidity due to preeclampsia varies between 3.8 and 12 per 1000 births. In Latin America, there are few reports on the subject, so the real magnitude of the problem remains unknown; there are only some studies from Brazil and Cuba [11].

Throughout the world, 25% of all maternal deaths occur in adolescent women. In Latin America, adolescent pregnancy is an independently associated factor conferring greater risk for adversities during pregnancy [12, 13]. In the United States, the maternal mortality rate due to preeclampsia-eclampsia is approximately 1 for every 100,000 live births. In Mexico, maternal mortality has decreased in the past six decades, whereby 1281 maternal deaths were registered in the year 2009, in women between the ages of 15 and 34 [14].

The main causes of death in pregnant women were:

1. Hypertensive disease induced by pregnancy (20.4%).

2. Obstetric hemorrhage (19%).

3. Sepsis (4.1%).

These percentages are five to ten times greater than those reported in industrialized nations or in those with more developed national health systems [15, 16].

6. Definitions of hypertensive states in pregnancy

According to the American College of Obstetricians and Gynecologists (ACOG) [17–19], the classification of hypertensive disorders in pregnancy is as follows:

Hypertensive disease induced by pregnancy:

- Preeclampsia
    - Mild
    - Severe
- Eclampsia

Chronic hypertension before pregnancy (any etiology).

Chronic hypertension and pregnancy-induced hypertension:

- Preeclampsia
- Eclampsia

6.1 Pregnancy-induced hypertensive disorders

Pregnancy-induced hypertension (PIH) is defined as the disorder that develops during gestation, delivery, or postpartum, characterized by elevated blood pressure values ≥140/90 mm Hg, accompanied by signs and symptoms allowing it to be classified according to its severity.

6.2 Preeclampsia

Preeclampsia refers to the presence of hypertension with values above those previously mentioned and proteinuria, in a pregnant female after the 20th week, after excluding hydatidiform mole or hydrops fetalis.

Arterial hypertension (AH) is diagnosed if the obtained values exceed, on two separate occasions and with at least 6 hours between each measurement, 140/90 mm Hg or if there is an increase in systolic arterial pressure (SAP) of at least 30 mm Hg or an increase in diastolic arterial pressure (DAP) of at least 15 mm Hg.

Proteinuria can be diagnosed with a urine test strip but must be confirmed with a quantitative method (urine sample or 24-hour urine).

Proteinuria must be above >300 mg in the urine collected in 24 hours or the protein: creatinine ratio must be ≥0.3.

6.3 Severe preeclampsia

Severe preeclampsia is defined as a systolic BP ≥160 mm Hg and/or a diastolic BP ≥110 mm Hg, if detected on two separate occasions, with a 6-hour difference, with proteinuria greater than 5 g/24 hours and no previous history of arterial hypertension, diabetic nephropathy, or renal disease.

HELLP syndrome is the acronym of hemolysis, elevated liver enzyme levels, and low platelet levels; this syndrome occurs in 10–20% of women with preeclampsia or eclampsia and is considered a severe form of the disease since it leads to increased mortality.

6.4 Eclampsia

It is defined as the presence of seizures or coma in a patient with preeclampsia, and that cannot be explained by another underlying cause.

6.5 Chronic hypertension

BP > 140/90 mm Hg before pregnancy or the same obtained values on two separate occasions prior to week 20 of gestation or persistent hypertension after the sixth week postpartum.

6.6 Chronic hypertension and pregnancy-induced hypertension

It is defined as an increase in SAP greater than 30 mm Hg or an increase greater than 15 mm Hg in DAP, on two separate occasions, prior to week 20 of gestation, initial proteinuria, and generalized edema.

6.7 Transient or late arterial hypertension

This is hypertension developing in the postpartum without previous preeclampsia; values return to baseline after the tenth day postpartum.

7. Physiopathology of preeclampsia

Preeclampsia is a syndrome that compromises all maternal organs and systems.

The etiology of hypertensive disorders in pregnancy remains to be identified since searching for their origin has led to an infinite number of hypotheses that encompass practically all maternal and fetal organs.

Its physiopathology has not been totally elucidated, and it is no different in the *adolescent* patient than in the rest of the affected population.

Several factors have been implicated in its physiopathology such as oxidative stress, the inflammatory response, abnormal circulatory adaptation, metabolic abnormalities, and even abnormalities in placental development, releasing circulating factors that interfere with vascular endothelial growth factor (VEGF) and placental growth factor (PGF).

Aside from the physiopathogenic factors to be discussed ahead, many factors predisposing to preeclampsia have been reported, such as extreme ages (very young or older), nulliparity, obesity, smoking, a history of preeclampsia in a previous pregnancy, etc. Other less studied factors include some infections, asthma, and the time period between pregnancies [20].

7.1 Systemic endothelial dysfunction

Endothelial abnormality leads to dysfunction in the control of muscle tone in blood vessels which, in turn, may cause hypertension, edema due to increased permeability, and also proteinuria.

Likewise, the abnormal expression of procoagulant factors by the endothelium favors the development of coagulopathy. All of these abnormalities injure target organs such as the kidney, the liver, the central nervous system, and the placenta. Women with previous vascular disease are at greater risk of developing preeclampsia, quite possibly a result of preestablished vascular injury.

7.1.1 First phase: abnormal placentation and placental ischemia

The placenta plays a pivotal role in the development of preeclampsia since it only develops in its presence and symptoms rapidly remit after delivery.

During the development of normal placentation, the cytotrophoblast invades the spiral arteries which leads to their remodeling; they will have low resistance and high elasticity or capacitance. This cytotrophoblastic vascular invasion not only affects the most superficial layers but reaches the muscle tunica. Trophoblast penetration has also been reported as incomplete and is not invasive in patients with preeclampsia; after complete remodeling of the spiral arteries, placental perfusion decreases. Although remodeling of the spiral arteries begins in the first trimester, it is not considered complete until weeks 18–20 of gestation.

Recently, great importance has been attributed to angiogenesis because of molecules such as VEGF, angiopectin, and other proteins in the ephrin family. The invasive trophoblast expresses VEGF, P1GF, VEGF, and their respective receptors. Likewise, in in vitro studies in which these signals were blocked, integrin alpha-1, a marker of pseudovasculogenesis, decreased alarmingly.

7.1.2 Second phase: systemic endothelial dysfunction

As previously mentioned, systemic endothelial dysfunction in these patients may explain all or almost all of the clinical signs, such as hypertension, proteinuria, or abnormalities in target organs such as the liver, the central nervous system, or the kidneys.

Among the various findings upholding this theory, we can mention the following:

- The plasma elevation in some biomarkers, such as fibronectin, factor VIII, and thrombomodulin, reflects endothelial cell injury in patients with preeclampsia.

- Vasodilation mediated by flow has also been reported in the vessels of women with preeclampsia, suggesting altered endothelial function.

- Decreased production of vasodilators such as prostacyclins or an increase in the production of angiotensin II also suggests endothelial injury.

- In these patients, renal biopsies show diffuse glomerular injury caused by glomerular endotheliosis.

- Likewise, the serum of women with preeclampsia has been shown to activate the endothelium in in vitro studies using endothelial cells from the umbilical veins.

An important factor for future consideration is that the increased concentrations of sFlt-1 generally precede, by 5 weeks, the development of clinical manifestations and appear to be most elevated in the initial phase of severe preeclampsia. However, neither PlGF nor VEGF, measured during gestation, appears to decrease prior to the onset of preeclampsia symptoms.

Most recently, decreases in urinary PIGF have been described before the development of preeclampsia. Some authors have speculated that sFlt-1 plays a beneficial role in fetal circulation and that preeclampsia is a reflection of a maladaptive effect of its release into the maternal circulation. Thus, in the setting of some spiral arterioles with increased resistance, vasoconstriction of the nonplacental maternal circulation would theoretically increase the cardiac output percentage reaching the placental sub-circulation. Although most cases of preeclampsia are sporadic, some authors suggest that genetics play a role in the development of this entity based on a series of findings:

- Primiparous women with a positive family history of preeclampsia have a two- to fivefold greater risk of developing preeclampsia than primiparous women without this history.

- In sisters with preeclampsia, the genetic imprint plays a major role in the development of the disease.

- Studies in women pregnant with males that were the result of a gestation with preeclampsia have greater probabilities of developing the disease in their pregnancies.

- Women who became pregnant with men whose previous partner had preeclampsia have greater probabilities of developing the disease if gestation with the previous partner was normotensive [20].

7.2 Preeclampsia-eclampsia in adolescents

Traditional references accept that the risk of preeclampsia-eclampsia in adolescents is twice that in the adult population. However, literature reviews are contradictory; while one group of authors refer to an increased risk of preeclampsia in adolescents [21], others detect no differences between these and adult pregnant women, as shown in **Table 2**.

Several studies and meta-analysis [22] detect a significant difference between pregnant adolescents and adult women, with up to 20% more preeclampsia events in pregnant adolescents than in adult women [23]; they actually report a greater risk of preeclampsia-eclapmsia in the group of adolescents between the ages of 13 and 16 when compared with women between the ages of 20 and 34, OR 2.97 (95%CI 1.62–5.42) [24], as well as lower frequencies of preeclampsia in adolescents (5%) vs. 1.5% in the adult group, and the difference was statistically significant, OR 3.66 (95%CI 1.67–7.72) [25].

Therefore, the frequency of preeclampsia in adolescents is currently different according to the studied population as a result of many factors such as prenatal care and body weight changes in pregnancy [26–29].

There is significant bias in observational studies that depend on the type of design and case identification; in these cases, no significant association is found suggesting an increased frequency of preeclampsia in pregnant adolescents, RR 0.88 (95%CI 95% 0.73–1.23). On the contrary, if we take into account follow-up studies, the pregnant adolescent is 23% less likely to develop preeclampsia when compared with pregnant women in other age ranges, RR 0.77 (95%CI 0.64–0.92).

Therefore, the available evidence suggests that adolescence is not a determining factor in the development of preeclampsia and eclampsia, but geographic area does appear to be an additional factor.

In a systematic review [30] describing pregnant adolescents that participated in integral prenatal care programs, they had a lower risk of developing pregnancy-induced hypertension (RR 0.59) than those following traditional prenatal care programs. This means that integral prenatal care programs focused on adolescents decrease the frequency of pregnancy-induced pregnancy by 41% [10].

Due to the heterogeneous presentations of preeclampsia in adolescents from different regions, age is probably not a determining factor but is rather associated to

Parra [38]	Under 19 year 13.5%			The prevalence is greater than 17–19 years before the age of 17 $p < 0.001$	
Zeck et al. [25]	5% in adolescents vs 1.5% in adults			OR 3.666 (1.627, 7.723)	
Tebeu et al. [24]	Risk of 13–16 vs 20–34 years			OR 2.974 (1.627, 5.427)	
Gronvik [22]	Meta-analysis			OR 3.52 (2.26, 5.48)	
Bostanci et al. [21]		Age of resolution $P < 0.001$	Number of appointments $P < 0.001$	Prevalence of preeclampsia $P < 0.001$	aOR $p < 0.001$
	Early adolescent 11–13 years	36 weeks	3.0	4.8%	1.14 (0.031, 0.63)
	Middle adolescent 14–16 years	37 weeks	4.78		
	Late adolescent 17–19 years	38 weeks	5.54	2.7%	0.44 (0.31, 0.63)
	Adult			5.9%	2.1 (1.51, 3.01)
Garmer [39]	Hypertensive disorders related with pregnancy $P = 0.99$				
	<20 years			20–34 years	
	8.7%			9.2%	
Azevedo et al. [6]	Hypertensive disorders in pregnancy			10%	

Table 2.
Prevalences of preeclampsia in adolescents.

other variables, such as excess weight, excessive weight gain during pregnancy, and inadequate prenatal care, among others.

Two factors warrant analysis in terms of the development of preeclampsia in pregnant adolescents; the first is its association with obesity. Obesity is currently considered an epidemic in which one of every four women in reproductive age is obese and over half of women between the ages of 20 and 39 have excess weight or obesity. Obesity has been reported to increase the risk of adverse maternofetal outcomes due to its association to and development of comorbidities such as gestational diabetes, fetal macrosomia, an increase in cesarean sections, and preeclampsia. Its genesis is the increase in oxidative stress; an increase in circulating pro-inflammatory biomarkers such as C-reactive protein, tumor necrosis factor-alpha, interleukin-6, and interleukin-8; the presence of dyslipidemia, insulin resistance, and abnormalities of endothelial function, all playing a role in the pathogenesis of preeclampsia [31].

Another factor leading to a poor maternal-perinatal outcome and that also increases the risk of preeclampsia is an inadequate nutrient intake, including calcium, zinc, vitamin C, vitamin E, and essential fatty acids. This factor has a doubly negative effect and results from the fact that adolescents are still growing, and during pregnancy, nutrients compete with the fetus for development, therefore leading to nutritional deficiencies [31].

As to the studies recommended in pregnant adolescents to screen for preeclampsia, there are currently no specific tests that can help establish a preclinical diagnosis, so the methods used in the general population are the only option:

1. First trimester combined test: markers (weight, blood pressure), ultrasound markers (uterine Doppler), and biochemical markers (PAPP-A, sFlt-1/PIGF).

2. Prophylactic aspirin before the 16th week of gestation in patients at greatest risk, based on an abnormal uterine Doppler in the first trimester.

3. In the second trimester, a uterine Doppler combined with other variables has a high negative predictive value.

Since there is no defined pattern in adolescent preeclampsia, its diagnosis and treatment must be the same as in the general population.

Therefore, the following recommendations have been established [32]:

In pregnant adolescents, screening, diagnostic, and therapeutic interventions should be similar to those applied in the rest of the population. **Level of evidence, moderate. Recommendation, strong.**

Care of pregnant adolescents must be provided in *ex profeso* clinics with complete, integral, and multidisciplinary programs to decrease maternal and perinatal risks, including pregnancy-induced hypertension. **Level of evidence, moderate. Recommendation, strong.**

Although there is no evidence on the beneficial effect of interventions used to curb weight gain during pregnancy, offering a medical evaluation and nutritional counseling is a good practice to recommend. **Level of evidence, low. Recommendation, strong.**

Every adolescent clinic must establish the incidence of preeclampsia and eclampsia in its patient population and determine which factors are associated to their development. **Level of evidence, low. Recommendation, strong.**

According to the diagnostic situation of preeclampsia and eclampsia in each adolescent clinic, screening, preventive, early detection, and therapeutic programs must be designed. **Level of evidence, moderate. Recommendation, strong.**

In adolescents with preeclampsia, the disease is generally manifested in the latter part of gestation, close to full-term delivery, so good prenatal care fosters a timely diagnosis of hypertensive disease in earlier stages and improves maternal and fetal outcomes. In the case of the induction of delivery, outcomes will also be improved by decreasing the need for cesarean delivery even in the cases of severe preeclampsia: the neonatal outcome also improves since age is not an influencing factor but disease severity is.

8. Long-term fetal complications in hypertensive mothers

Follow-up of the offspring of mothers with any pregnancy-associated hypertensive state [33] has shown that by age 7, their systolic blood pressure is increased although within normal parameters—SBP of 104 mm Hg (95%CI 101–106 vs. SBP 99 mm Hg, 95%CI 99–100, $p = 0.001$)—and this cardiometabolic injury is evident from the age of 2 years.

This abnormality is only observed in full-term births and not in premature offspring; a posited explanation is that the stress caused by preterm delivery protects the fetus from sequelae.

Another consequence observed in the offspring of hypertensive mothers is the development of hypertension and cerebral vascular disease when these children reach adulthood. Also, their risk of developing hypertension increases if their body mass index is elevated, and this has been observed since the ages of 4–10, even if the mother had hypertension with no proteinuria; the presence of elevated liver enzymes or thrombocytopenia has also been associated with hypertension in young offspring [34, 35].

Fetal changes due to maternal hypertension have been associated with genetic and environmental mechanisms that condition modifications in fetal programming [36]. Among the effects caused by preeclampsia, one hypothesis suggests that superficial invasion of spiral arteries leads to fetal malnutrition. Changes in fetal programming may also involve abnormalities in the inflammatory response and endothelial dysfunction associated with preeclampsia.

An important point in this description of long-term sequelae in the offspring of pregnant adolescents is that they are not modified by age.

9. Points to remember

- Adolescent pregnancy is a very important biopsychosocial event, a public health issue, and a continuous social reflection.
- Hypertensive problem associated with pregnancy including the period of adolescence is another public health issue; its prevalence in the worldwide is around 10% of all pregnancies.
- Preeclampsia in adolescents refers to a relatively common hypertensive disorder during pregnancy that develops progressively. Its cause remains unknown, and it frequently leads to severe maternal and perinatal complications.
- The incidence is broad since it depends on various aspects such as geographic location, race, nutritional or immunological factors, and associated comorbidities.
- Traditional references accept that the risk of preeclampsia-eclampsia in adolescents is twice that in the adult population, but in recent studies including meta-analysis, the presence of preeclampsia in pregnant adolescents varies from a 20% more frequent and specifically in the group of 13–16 years (OR 2.97, 95% CI 1.62–5.42) to 23% less. Therefore, the available evidence suggests that adolescence is not a determining factor in the development of preeclampsia and eclampsia, but geographic area does appear to be an additional factor.
- Two other determinants of risk factor for developing preeclampsia in pregnant adolescent are obesity and inadequate nutrient intake (calcium, zinc, vitamin C, vitamin E, and essential fatty acids).
- In adolescents with preeclampsia, the disease is generally manifested in the latter part of gestation, close to full-term delivery.
- A good prenatal care fosters timely diagnosis of hypertensive disease in earlier stages and improves maternal and fetal outcomes.

Author details

Sergio Rosales-Ortiz*, Olivia Sánchez Rodríguez, Mario Borbolla-Ramos and Karen D. García-Pérez
Hospital de Gineco Obstetricia No. 4 "Luis Castelazo Ayala", Mexican Social Security Institute, México City, Mexico

*Address all correspondence to: dr.sergiorosalesortiz@gmail.com

References

[1] Mundial de la Infancia. La adolescencia una época de oportunidades.pdf. 2011. Available from: http://www.unicef.org/bolivia/UNICEF-eSTADO

[2] Organización Panamericana de Salud. La salud de los adolescentes y jóvenes en las Américas. Washington: OPS/OMS; 1996

[3] Futterman D, Chabon B, Hoffman ND. HIV and AIDS in adolescents. Pediatric Clinics of North America. 2000;**47**(1):171-188

[4] Carvalho RC, Campos H, Bruno ZV, Mota RM. Fatores preditivos de hipertensão gestacional em adolescentes primíparas: Análise do pré-natal, da MAPA e da microalbuminúria. Arquivos Brasileiros de Cardiologia. 2006;**87**(4):487-495

[5] Chalem E, Mitsuhiro SS, Ferri CP, et al. Gravidez na adolescência: Perfil sócio-demográfico e comportamental de uma população da periferia de São Paulo, Brasil. Cadernos de Saúde Pública. 2007;**23**(1):177-186

[6] Azevedo WF, Diniz MB, Fonseca ES, et al. Complications in adolescent pregnancy. Einstein. 2015;**13**(4):618-626

[7] Widman L, Choukas-Bradley S, Helms SW. Sexual communication between early adolescents and their dating partners, parents, and best friends. Journal of Sex Research. 2014;**51**(7):731-741

[8] Ruoti M, Ruoti A, et al. Sexualidad y embarazo en adolescentes. Instituto de Investigaciones de Ciencias de Salud. Paraguay: Universidad de Asunción; 12 April 1992

[9] Elster AB. The Medical and psychosocial impact of a comprehensive care on adolescent pregnancy and parenthood. Journal of the American Medical Association. 1987;**258**:1187-1192

[10] Mueller T et al. Teen pregnancy prevention: Implementation of a multicomponent, community-wide approach. The Journal of Adolescent Health. 2017;**60**:9-17

[11] Bhattacharya S, Campbell DM. The incidence of severe complications of preeclampsia. Hypertension Pregnancy. 2005;**24**:181-190

[12] Al-Suleiman SA, Qutub HO, Rahman J, et al. Obstetric admissions to the intensive care unit: A 12-year review. Archives of Gynecology and Obstetrics. 2006;**274**(1):4-8

[13] Osinaike BB, Amanor-Boadu SD, Sanusi AA. Obstetric intensive care: A developing country experience. The Internet Journal of Anesthesiology. 2006;**10**(2):1-5

[14] Loverro G, Pansini V, Greco P, et al. Indications and outcome for intensive care unit admission during puerperium. Archives of Gynecology and Obstetrics. 2001;**265**:195-198

[15] Conde-Agudelo A, Belizán JM, Lammers C. Maternal-perinatal morbidity and mortality associated with adolescent pregnancy in Latin America: Cross-sectional study. American Journal of Obstetrics and Gynecology. 2005;**192**:342-349

[16] World Health Organization. Maternal Mortality in 2008: Estimates Developed by WHO, UNICEF, UNFPA, and the World Bank. Geneva: World Health Organization; 2009

[17] American College of Obstetricians and Gynecologists. Task force on hypertension in pregnancy. Hypertension in Pregnancy. Obstetrics and Gynecology. 2013;**122**:1122-1131

[18] Report of the National High Blood Pressure Education Program. working group on high blood pressure in pregnancy. American Journal of Obstetrics and Gynecology 2000;**183**:s1-s22

[19] Leaños-Miranda A, Márquez-Acosta J, Romero-Arauz F, et al. Protein: Creatinine ratio in random urine samples is a reliable marker of increased 24-hour protein excretion in hospitalized women with hypertensive disorders of pregnancy. Clinical Chemistry. 2007;**53**:1623-1628

[20] Curiel E, Prieto MA, Mora J. Factores relacionados con el desarrollo de preeclampsia. Revisión de la bibliografía. Clínica e Investigación en Ginecología y Obstetricia. 2008;**35**(3):87-97

[21] Bostanci EE, Abide YC, Ozkaya E, et al. Maternal-fetal outcome associated with adolescent pregnancy in a tertiary referral center: A cross-sectional study. Ginekologia Polska. 2017;**88**(12):674-678

[22] Gronvik T, Fossgard S. Complications associated with adolescent childbearing in Sub-Saharan Africa: A systematic literature review and meta-analysis. PLoS One. 2018;**13**(9):0204327

[23] Adeyinka DA, Oladimeji TI, Odekanbi TI, et al. Outcome of adolescent pregnancies in southwestern Nigeria: A case-control study. The Journal of Maternal-Fetal and Neonatal Medicine. 2010;**23**(8):785-789

[24] Tebeu PM, Foumane P, Mbu R, et al. Risk factors for hypertensive disorders in pregnancy: A report from the Maroua Regional Hospital, Cameroon. Journal of Reproduction and Infertility. 2011;**12**(3):227-234

[25] Zeck W, Wilkinson J, Obure J, et al. Comparison of obstetrical risk in adolescent primiparas at tertiary referral centres in Tanzania and Austria. The Journal of Maternal-Fetal and Neonatal Medicine. 2010;**23**(12):1470-1474

[26] Karabulut A, Ozkan S, Bozkurt AI, et al. Perinatal outcomes and risk factors in adolescent and advanced age pregnancies: Comparison with normal reproductive age women. Journal of Obstetrics and Gynaecology. 2013;**33**(4):346-350

[27] Leppalahti S, Gissler M, Mentula M, et al. Is teenage pregnancy an obstetric risk in a welfare society? A population-based study in Finland, from 2006 to 2011. BMJ Open. 2013;**3**(8):003225

[28] Hoque M, Hoque S. Comparison of perinatal and obstetrics outcomes among early adolescents, late adolescents and adult pregnant women from rural South Africa. East African Journal of Public Health. 2010;**7**(2):171-176

[29] Thaithae S, Thato R. Obstetric and perinatal outcomes of teenage pregnancies in Thailand. Journal of Pediatric and Adolescent Gynecology. 2011;**24**(6):342-346

[30] Scholl TO, Hediger ML, Belsky DH. Prenatal care and maternal health during adolescent pregnancy: A review and meta-analysis. The Journal of Adolescent Health. 1994;**15**:444-456

[31] Aliyu MH, Luke S, Kristense S, et al. Joint effect of obesity and teenage pregnancy on the risk of preeclampsia: A population-based study. Journal of Adolescent Health. 2010;**46**:77-82

[32] Lira PJ, Oviedo CH. Evaluación de riesgo materno-infantil en el control prenatal en adolescentes. Guía de práctica clínica. Colegio Mexicano de Especialistas en Ginecología y Obstetricia (COMEGO). 2014:380-395

[33] Murguia RM, Landn MB, Varner MW, et al. Pregnancy-associated hypertension and offspring cardiometabolic health. Obstetrics and Gynecology. 2018;**131**(2):313-321

[34] Davis EF, Lazdam M, Lwandowski AJ, et al. Cardiovascular risk factors in children and young adults born to preeclamptic pregnancies: A systematic review. Pediatrics. 2012;**129**:1552-1561

[35] Zimmet P, Alberti KG, Kaufman F, et al. The metabolic syndrome in children and adolescent an IDF consensus report. Pediatric Diabetes. 2007;**8**:299-306

[36] Barker DJ, Larsen G, Osmond C, et al. The placental origins of sudden cardiac death. International Journal of Epidemiology. 2012;**41**:1394-1399

[37] Kawakita T, Wilson K, Grantz KL, et al. Adverse maternal and neonatal outcomes in adolescent pregnancy. Journal of Pediatric and Adolescent Gynecology. 2016;**29**(2):130-136

[38] Parra-Pingel PE, Quisguiña-Avellán LA, Hidalgo L, Chdraui P, Pérez-López FR. Pregnancy outcomes in younger and older adolescent mothers with severe preeclampsia. Adolescent Health, Medicine and Therapeutics. 2017;**8**:81-86

[39] Garmer AJ, Robertson A, Thomton C, et al. Adolescent perinatal outcoms in South West Sidney, Australia. Mayo Clinic Proceedings: Innovations, Quality & Outcomes. 2018;**2**(1):10-15